RESPITE FOR CAREGIVERS OF ALZHEIMER PATIENTS
Research and Practice

M. Powell Lawton, Ph.D., has been Director of Research at the Philadelphia Geriatric Center for 27 years. He is an Adjunct Professor of Human Development at the Pennsylvania State University and Professor of Psychiatry at the Medical College of Pennsylvania, and he has a doctorate in clinical psychology from Columbia University. He has done research in the environmental psychology of later life, in assessment of the aged, the psychological well-being of older people, caregiving stress, and has conducted evaluative studies of programs for the aged and for the mentally ill.

Dr. Lawton has served as President of the American Psychological Association's Division on Adult Development and Aging. He was member of the 1971 White House Conference on Aging. He is the author of *Environment and Aging* and *Planning and Managing Housing for the Elderly*, as well as the editor of other books.

His awards include the Kleemeier Award of the Gerontological Society of America, the Distinguished Contribution Award of the American Psychological Association's Division on Adult Development and Aging, the Career Award of the Environmental Design Research Association, the Ollie Randall Award of the Northeastern Gerontological Society, and the Annual Award of the Philadelphia Society of Clinical Psychologists.

Elaine M. Brody, M.S.W., Sc.D. (Hon.), was Associate Director of Research at the Philadelphia Geriatric Center and Director of the Department of Human Resources. She is currently Senior Research Consultant at the organization, and is Clinical Professor of Psychiatry in the Department of Psychiatry at the Medical College of Pennsylvania and Adjunct Associate Professor of Social Work in Psychiatry in the School of Medicine at the University of Pennsylvania. Her most recent book is *Women in the Middle: Their Parent Care Years* (Springer Publishing Company, New York).

Mrs. Brody is a past President of the Gerontological Society of America. She received an honorary doctorate, D.Sc., from the Medical College of Pennsylvania in April 1987 and has been elected as a Distinguished Scholar of the National Academies of Practice. Among the awards she has received are the 1985 Brookdale Award of the Gerontological Society of America and the 1983 Donald P. Kent Award of the Gerontological Society of America. Mrs. Brody was selected as a Woman of the Year, *Ms* (magazine), January 1986. Her publications include five books, numerous book chapters, and over 200 journal articles. Mrs. Brody has directed 15 federally financed research studies in the field of gerontology.

Avalie Saperstein, A.C.S.W., L.S.W., is Director of the Department of Social Services and Therapeutic Activities and Director of the Department of Community Services at the Philadelphia Geriatric Center.

She has been instrumental in establishing innovative community-based programs and has been involved in counseling and educating individuals and organizations that provide services to the elderly.

Ms. Saperstein is a member of the Gerontological Society of America, the National Association of Social Workers and the Academy of Certified Social Workers. She holds a Master's of Social Work degree from the University of Washington.

RC
523
.L38
1991

RESPITE FOR CAREGIVERS OF ALZHEIMER PATIENTS

Research and Practice

M. Powell Lawton
Elaine M. Brody
Avalie R. Saperstein

SPRINGER PUBLISHING COMPANY

New York

GOSHEN COLLEGE LIBRARY
GOSHEN, INDIANA

Copyright © 1991 by Springer Publishing Company

All rights reserved

No part of this publication may be reproduced, stored in a
retrieval system, or transmitted in any form or by any means,
electronic, mechanical, photocopying, recording, or otherwise,
without the prior permission of Springer Publishing Company, Inc.

Springer Publishing Company, Inc.
536 Broadway
New York, NY 10012-3955

91 92 93 94 95 / 5 4 3 2 1

Library of Congress Cataloging-in-Publication Data

Lawton, M. Powell (Mortimer Powell), 1923–
    Respite for caregivers of Alzheimer patients : research and
practice / M. Powell Lawton, Elaine M. Brody, Avalie R. Saperstein.
        p. cm.
    Based on results of a study conducted by the Philadelphia
Geriatric Center (PGC).
    Includes bibliographical references and index.
    ISBN 0-8261-6610-5
    1. Alzheimer's disease—Patients—Respite care. 2. Alzheimer's
disease—Patients—Family relationships. I. Brody, Elaine M.
II. Saperstein, Avalie R. III. Philadelphia Geriatric Center.
IV. Title.
    [DNLM: 1. Alzheimer's Disease. 2. Health Services for the Aged—
organization & administration. 3. Home Nursing. 4. Respite Care.
WM 220 L425r]
RC523.L38   1991
362.1'98976831—dc20
DNLM/DLC
for Library of Congress   91-4615
                                                             CIP

Printed in the United States of America

Contents

Introduction

In recent years, respite service for caregivers has gained widespread attention as one of a number of strategies that seem to foster community care for the disabled aged. Though there is no generally accepted definition of that service, the United States Department of Health and Human Services describes it as "short term inpatient or outpatient care delivered to an elderly person in lieu of his or her regular support" (U.S. Department of Health and Human Services, January 1981).

The view of respite as having potential for ameliorating the strains on family caregivers is usually coupled with the program goal of reducing the economic costs of care by preventing or delaying nursing home admissions. Respite also has emerged consistently as the top priority unmet need expressed by caregivers. This book describes and reports the findings from a respite service project conducted by the Philadelphia Geriatric Center (PGC) that was designed specifically for families caring for victims of Alzheimer's disease and related disorders. Moreover, implications for planning and delivering respite programs are detailed, based on the project's operating experiences as well as on its research findings.

The PGC respite service study was made possible by funding from two foundations. The demonstration project, *A Multiser-*

vice Respite Program for Family Caregivers of Patients with Alzheimer's Disease, was financed by the John A. Hartford Foundation of New York, and its companion research study, *Respite Care for the Alzheimer's Disease Patient and Family: A Research Evaluation* was funded by the Pew Charitable Trusts (The Medical Trust) of Philadelphia. The study responded to widespread concern about the increasing number of people with Alzheimer's disease* and related disorders, the well-documented negative effects of providing care on many of their family caregivers, and the need for the latter to be afforded temporary relief from the provision of ongoing care. Because such patients are over-represented in nursing homes, the economic as well as the social costs of their care are high. The major goals of the project, therefore, were to evaluate the potential of respite service to improve the well-being of caregivers and to determine whether the economic costs of care could be reduced by delaying or avoiding institutionalization.

For purposes of the project, *respite care* was defined as *any service or group of services designed to provide temporary periods of relief and/or rest for caregivers away from the patient.* Such a flexible and inclusive definition made it possible to tailor highly individualized programs to the needs of each participating family.

The Philadelphia Geriatric Center was deemed an appropriate auspice for the study because of its demonstrated capacity to deliver or mobilize a wide-range of services and because of its long-standing commitment to Alzheimer's patients and their families. In brief, the PGC is a nonprofit multiservice agency that serves about 1200 older people who live on its campus in a variety of facilities, including a fully accredited geriatric hospital, skilled and intermediate care nursing homes, and high-rise service supported apartment buildings. The PGC also serves thousands of older people who live in their own

---

*The term Alzheimer's disease will be used throughout this book to describe irreversible senile dementia, the main forms of which are Alzheimer's disease and multi-infarct dementia. The symptoms of those ailments are similar and, therefore, the practical problems and social needs for care are the same.

homes or the homes of relatives in the greater Philadelphia area. Its programs and services (both in- and out-patient) have always focused on caregiving families as well as on the older people themselves. For example, among the community services focusing on Alzheimer's patients and their families was a project to develop and staff family support groups. Thus, the essential program elements of the projected respite service were already in place at the PGC—specifically, nursing facilities, a hospital, and day care.

For a quarter of a century, the PGC has specialized in the care of and research about older people with Alzheimer's disease. In 1964 when professional and scientific interest was virtually nonexistent, the PGC convened the first international conference focusing on dementia (Lawton & Lawton, 1965). Innovative service and research activities continued through the years. Among those activities were studies of the treatment of "excess disabilities" of Alzheimer's patients and of appropriate institutional environments for their care, activity therapy to improve the quality of their lives and elevate their functioning levels, counseling groups for families of afflicted older people in the PGC nursing home, and support and counseling for family members providing community care. One outcome of the research was the building of a 120 bed facility specifically designed for Alzheimer's patients, the Sley Pavilion of the Weiss Institute, which opened in 1974. At present, plans are being completed for a center for the study and treatment of Alzheimer's Disease, unique in that it will combine patient care and research for the benefit of Alzheimer's sufferers and their families.

The Philadelphia Geriatric Center respite project involved the offering of all known forms of such care, organizing them into a system with the capability of responding to changing needs of the patient and family. The family was thereby helped to overcome both system and psychological barriers to use of the services. Thus, operating the project afforded a great deal of practical experience in developing, mobilizing, and delivering care, in forging linkages to other existing services in the community, and in enabling families to avail themselves to the help offered. This book presents not only the research aspects and findings of the study, but also the processes and principles involved in making respite service work. Therefore, a liberal amount of case material is used illustratively.

Chapter 1 of this book offers background information about the place of respite care in the larger long-term care service system. A review of the literature on respite care is also included. Chapter 2 describes the respite program that was offered as the experimental intervention, the kinds of services offered, the planning process, and the barriers to utilization. Chapters 3 through 5 describe the respite-service research and its major results. Chapter 6 considers both the research-based and experimental knowledge gained from this demonstration. This chapter is designed for practitioners, with particular regard for the many problems of administering such a program. The final chapter provides a summary and some conclusions meant to stimulate future thought, research, and practice.

Although the study and findings described focused on families of Alzheimer's disease patients, much of the material presented is applicable to respite service for families caring for disabled elderly with other diagnoses. The research design, for example, may inform those planning controlled studies of other service interventions. The psychological and service system barriers to service utilization and the counseling techniques have general applicability, as do the planning principles described in Chapter 6.

In summary, this book is a resource for operating respite programs, with many of its major principles being based on solid research findings. The authors' hope is that the ability of research and practice to enrich one another has been documented.

Acknowledgments

The service program and research required a large and devoted staff, most of whom cannot be thanked individually within the page limits of this volume. Special thanks, however, are due to Miriam Grimes, Project Director for the Research; Sandra diGiambattista and Allen Glicksman, computer and statistical advisors. Karen Reever and a group of dedicated service workers and interviewers delivered the respite services and collected the data. Finally, Anita Roffman, Bernice Albert, and Denise Boothman provided support skills in the preparation of the manuscript.

The support of the John A. Hartford Foundation entailed initial stimulation and long-term encouragement from John Billings, Ina Guzman, and Laura Robbins. Similarly, Brent Roehrs of the Pew Charitable Trusts was extraordinarily helpful in keeping the project moving. We are very grateful to these people and the administration of the two foundations.

Respite Services as an Element of the Long-Term Care System

1

Care of the uniquely disadvantaged older people who suffer from Alzheimer's disease or a related disorder presents extra-ordinary difficulties for families. Indeed, dementia is probably the most socially disruptive of all ailments. Concern about the severe strains experienced by family caregivers is being ex-pressed in part by the groundswell of attention to ways of providing them with some relief. Respite services top the list of services desired by professionals and the families themselves.

Though other demonstration respite programs had been mounted, the project described in this book was one of the first to be conceptualized as a randomized experiment. An earlier study had recruited caregivers explicitly for a respite study and assigned them to four experimental conditions and one control group (Montgomery, 1988). Of the 632 research participants in the study described in this book, half (the Experimental group) were offered respite and half (the Control group) were not. (The design of the research will be described fully in Chapter 3.)

In brief, the major aims of the research were to determine the effects of respite service on family caregivers; to identify the forms of respite they chose and preferred; to estimate the nature and number of different types of respite services required by a population of a given size; and to determine the effects of respite on utilization of other services and on rates of nursing home placement. In addition, operation of the program offered to the experimental group was expected to yield qualitative information about families' reasons for use or nonuse of the services and the needs that were served in doing so.

This chapter will present background information: data on the prevalence of Alzheimer's disease, the costs of care, service utilization by that population, and the effects of caring on family members. The literature on demonstrations of respite will be reviewed.

ALZHEIMER'S DISEASE AND OTHER FORMS OF DEMENTIA

The growth in the population of victims of Alzheimer's disease is due to two phases of the demographic revolution that occurred in this century. First, the number and proportion of older people in the United States has increased dramatically, rising from 4% of the total population in 1900 (3 million people) to 11.9% in 1984 (about 28.5 million people). Second, the elderly population has increased unevenly, with the oldest segment increasing most rapidly. This trend will continue: by the year 2000, the number of people 65 to 74 will increase by 23%, those 75 to 84 will increase by 57% and those 85 and over will almost double. Because the prevalence of severe dementia rises steeply with age—increasing from about 1% of those who are 65–74 to 7% of those 75 to 84, and to 25% of those 85 or over (Gurland & Cross, 1986)—it is clear that the future will see a major increase in prevalence. That projection could be upset, of course, if there should be a major biomedical breakthrough that prevents or ameliorates the disease.

Though estimates vary because of differing clinical criteria, the median of a number of single-community prevalence studies indicates that about 4% of older people living outside of institutions suffer from moderate to severe forms of dementia and related conditions. The most recent report by the Office of Technology Assessment (OTA) states that 1.5 million Americans suffer from severe dementia and another 1 to 5 million have mild or moderate cases (U.S. Congress, Office of Technology Assessment, 1987). Recent epidemiological studies suggest that the proportion may be even higher—that more than 11% of the elderly may suffer from underlying Alzheimer's disease (Cornoni-Huntley et al., 1985; Pfeffer, Afifi, & Chance, 1987). By the year 2040, the number of victims of severe dementia is projected to exceed 5 million Americans (Report of the Advisory Panel of Alzheimer's Disease, 1989).

To the number of noninstitutionalized victims of Alzheimer's must be added the number who live in institutions. The most recent national data show that in 1985 approximately 1.3 million persons, almost 5% of all Americans 65 years of age and over, were in institutions at any one time. Of those, 63% were disoriented or memory impaired—defined as being unable to remember dates or time, unable to identify familiar locations or people, unable to recall important aspects of recent events, or unable to make judgments (National Center for Health Statistics, 1987).

Functional disabilities in Activities of Daily Living (ADL) and Instrumental Activities of Daily Living (IADL), usually in conjunction with the absence of or decline in social supports, account for most admissions to nursing homes. Alzheimer's victims are not only characterized by multiple deficits in functioning, but present extraordinary management difficulties and cause social disruption in caregivers' lives. Thus, Alzheimer's constitutes a major social problem as well as an increasing public health problem and an important medical issue. It is estimated that the ailment is now the fifth greatest cause of mortality (Katzman & Karasu, 1975) because of secondary factors such as failure of ability to swallow and poor resistance to infection, as well as through primary brain atrophy.

The cost of care for Senile Dementia of the Alzheimer Type (SDAT) must be calculated both economically in dollars and socially in terms of the emotional and other burdens on caregivers. Estimates of the total annual cost for care of demented individuals, including costs of diagnosis, treatment, nursing home care and lost wages, range from $24 billion to $48 billion (U.S. Congress, OTA, 1987, p. 17). The annual cost of nursing home care for all residents is $38.9 billion (U.S. Congress, OTA, 1987, p. 18) and it is estimated that about 57% of nursing home residents have "chronic brain syndrome" (U.S. Department of Health and Human Services, 1981). (Estimates of the proportions of residents with dementia vary from study to study according to the different criteria used, but always are more than half.)

Much attention has been given to comparing the costs of nursing home care and community care for disabled older people. One review stated, ". . . the cost-effectiveness of home care for many long-term care patients and the relationships of home care to reduced institutionalization rates has not been demonstrated either in the United States or abroad" (Grana, 1983). Recent demonstrations have failed to yield consistent evidence of cost savings in offering community-based service alternatives to nursing home care (Capitman, 1989; Zawadski, 1983). For older people as disabled as those in institutions, the expense of home care is equal to or greater than that of institutional care (e.g., see Comptroller General, 1977a; Fox & Clauser, 1980; Palmer, 1983). In a study of the Cleveland area (Comptroller General of the United States 1977b), dollar costs to the community for noninstitutionalized people were lower because a substantial portion of those costs was borne by the family. Large-scale experiments providing case managed services (such as homemakers, personal care and home-delivered meals) did not reduce institutional costs because most of the elderly participants would have stayed in the community with or without the added services (Kemper, Applebaum, & Harrigan, 1987).

ALZHEIMER FAMILIES' USE OF FORMAL AND INFORMAL SERVICES

Despite the evidence, however, many of the community-based long-term care alternatives may be of marginal relevance to families when their relative has Alzheimer's disease. One rationale for the respite project, therefore, was that respite has been an inadequately tried form of community support that would be of benefit in taking occasional pressure off primary caregivers and their families and might, at the same time, lower the cost of institutional care to society. Moreover, though there had been many demonstration projects of respite care, the project was unique in that it had a careful, multifaceted control group design.

While definitive data are not available about the amount of formal, publicly financed services received by noninstitutionalized Alzheimer's patients, they probably receive little such service. The National Health Interview Survey, for example, found that in the year prior to the survey 1% of all older persons used homemaker services, 3% received care from visiting nurses, and about 2% used home health aides; utilization of adult day care and telephone call-check services was even lower (Stone, 1986). Rates of utilization were consistently lower for those older people living with others than for those living alone. Because the vast majority of Alzheimer's patients live with others, the evidence suggests that they are a low service group. The 1982 Long-Term Care Survey sponsored by the Department of Health and Human Services also showed the relatively small role played by formal services in helping the disabled aged. About 15% of all "helper days" for disabled older people living in the community came from formal sources, the rest being provided by the informal system (Doty, Liu, & Wiener, 1985). Only 4% of severely disabled older people received any subsidized services at all, with most formal help received being purchased by the older person or family.

In short, families provide the bulk of care to noninstitutionalized older people, including those with Alzheimer's disease: personal care (bathing, dressing, feeding, etc.), instrumental services (shopping, transportation, household maintenance), medically related care (such as injections and medication), continuous supervision, and emotional support (Brody, Johnson, & Fulcomer, 1982; Cantor, 1980; Sussman, 1976; Comptroller General of the U.S., 1977a; U.S. Public Health Service,

1972). When the patient is married, the spouse (aided by adult children) gives most of the care; adult children (primarily daughters) provide most of the care for those among the more than 9 million widowed elderly who need it (Gurland, Dean, Gurland, & Cook, 1978; Litman, 1971; Shanas, 1961; Stehouwer, 1968). In the 1982 Long-Term Care Survey, adult daughters provided more than half the care received by severely disabled older people (that is, those in need of help with ADL) (Stone, Cafferata, & Sangl, 1987).

Because people afflicted with Alzheimer's disease are generally the *very* old, their caregivers are most often either elderly themselves (when the patient is a spouse or a sibling) or in late middle age (when the patient is a parent), with their energies and strength depleted accordingly. The nature and symptoms of Alzheimer's disease often make it necessary for adult children to share their homes with such patients. Some caregivers are unable to leave their homes for weeks or months at a time.

Though concern has been expressed to the effect that service provision encourages the withdrawal of family care, that notion is not supported by the research evidence (see, for example, Kemper, Brown et al., 1987). To the contrary, services to caregiving families have been shown to strengthen and supplement family services, rather than to substitute for them (Horowitz & Dobrof, 1982; Zimmer & Mellor, 1981). Though family care is a major factor enabling older people to avoid institutionalization, prolonged, unrelieved, and unrelenting strain on caregivers often leads to the "point of no return" at which institutionalization of the parent or spouse become unavoidable (see Brody, 1987 for review).

Caregiver Strain

Despite the difficulties of providing care, the literature attests to the strong wish of many families to continue to care for their older relatives. Though there is definitive evidence that families have behaved very responsibly in caring for afflicted elderly people, Alzheimer's disease has been shown to be a strong predictor of caregiver strain (see Brody, 1987; Horowitz, 1985 for review). The symptoms of the ailment are uniquely distressing: confusion, poor memory, disorientation, diminished judgment, changes in intellectual functioning, wandering, behavior disturbances such as agitation and irritability, unpredictable emotional reactions, and disturbed sleep. Caregivers' burdens are increased by the need for constant surveillance and by the loss of the patient as a person who can communicate with them, relate to them, and provide feedback and appreciation.

Beginning with the classic Grad and Sainsbury (1966) research in the 1960s, research investigations have identified the care of mentally impaired older people as the most stressful to caregivers. Most of the symptoms found to be predictive of caregiver strain are characteristic of many Alzheimer's patients—incontinence and the need for considerable help because of multiple deficits in ADL, for example. Caring for a demented person has been found to be more damaging to family relationships and to the mental well-being of the primary caregiver than when the patient is physically disabled (Noelker & Poulshock, 1982). It is not the dementia per se that so often produces stress, however, but the disruptive behavioral manifestations of that ailment (Deimling & Bass, 1986; Horowitz, 1985).

Among the social and mental health costs to caregivers are: isolation; emotional problems (such as anxiety, depression, guilt, and insomnia); restrictions on family social and household activities; strained family relationships; exhaustion; despair; loneliness; loss of time from work; and economic problems (Archbold, 1978; Brody, Kleban, Lawton, & Silverman, 1987; Fengler & Goodrich, 1979; Grad & Sainsbury, undated; Lang & Brody, 1983; Newman, 1976). In turn, such problems can affect the care given to the older person (Gibson, 1982).

Sharing a household with a disabled older person is a strong predictor of strain. While mildly demented individuals may begin by remaining in their own homes, such arrangements cannot be sustained as the ailment progresses; virtually all noninstitutionalized Alzheimer's patients ultimately live with a caregiver.

A study by George (1984a) found that, in comparison to the general population, caregivers of Alzheimer's patients experienced more stress, took more prescription psychotropic drugs, participated in fewer social and recreational activities, and reported three times as many stress symptoms. Female caregivers (wives and daughters) were worse off than males on all of those effects. While spouse caregivers were more likely to use psychotropic drugs, to have financial problems, and to give up leisure, the filial caregivers (most of whom were daughters) reported higher levels of stress and unhappiness. An interesting finding from the George study was that overall levels of well-being did not differ for support group participants and nonparticipants. The support group participants did have more knowledge about Alzheimer's disease and about community services, however, and had fewer feelings that no one understands what one is experiencing in caregiving situations (George, 1986).

Data from a study of working and nonworking daughter caregivers also speak to the effects on the lives and well-being of those caring for a parent with Alzheimer's disease (Brody et al., 1987). Reports of depression among working daughters were related to having elderly parents with poor cognitive functioning and worry about being able to meet those parents' future needs. Moreover, more than one-fourth of nonworking daughters had quit their jobs in order to take care of their disabled parents and a similar proportion of the working daughters were "conflicted" in that they had reduced their working hours and/or were considering quitting because of parent care. The parents of both of those subgroups of women had poorer cognitive functioning than the mothers of the other daughters in the study and the daughters reported more problems and life-style disruptions. Data from the 1982 Long Term Care Survey (Stone et al., 1987) indicate that some spouses of disabled older people and sons (though to a lesser extent) also quit their jobs to take care of the impaired relatives. Virtually nothing is known about the opportunity costs incurred by those family members, though in the Brody study those who quit their jobs were the ones with the lowest family incomes.

Most reports about negative effects on caregivers' physical health derive from self-reports. Recently, however, a research group at the Ohio State University College of Medicine used objective physiologic measures in comparing family caregivers for Alzheimer's patients with matched subjects (Kiecolt-Glaser et al., 1987). It was demonstrated that the impact of the chronic stress on such caregivers resulted in lower levels of im-munological adaptations that may account for their greater susceptibility to physical health problems.

Taken together, the accumulated findings suggest that care of the demented patient is the most difficult form of family help, produces the most strain for caregivers, interferes the most with the caregivers' work lives, and has the most negative effects on family relationships and life styles. The proliferation of support groups for families of Alzheimer's patients and the publication of several books offering information and counsel to them (Cohen & Eisdorfer, 1986; Mace & Rabins, 1981; Safford, 1986) also attest to the severe problems such caregivers experience. An intriguing sidelight about caregiving adult children is that daughters experience more stress than sons. (For related discussion see Brody, 1990.)

Family Care After Nursing Home Placement

The number of demented older people who live in the community is equaled by the number who live in nursing homes. They are overrepresented in nursing homes, constituting about three-fifths of the total nursing-home population. Patients with Alzheimer's disease are the ones likely to need the most time consuming care whether they reside in the community (Mace & Rabins, 1981) or in the nursing home (Brody, Lawton, & Liebowitz, 1984). Community care is often described as a less costly "alternative" than nursing home care, but it is not cheaper in dollars and does not avoid nursing home placement for severely impaired people such as Alzheimer's patients (Weissert, 1985).

The special form of family caregiving that occurs after nursing home placement takes place has been given little attention.

It has long been known that the characteristics of the family are as influential as the characteristics of the older person as determinants of institutionalization (see Brody, 1985 for review). Specifically, while those in institutions are older, more disabled mentally and physically, and predominantly female, they also have fewer family supports than their counterparts who live in the community. The role of the family in maintaining older people in the community is highlighted by the fact that, in contrast to those who live in the community, only 16% of the institutionalized aged were married at the time of admission (65% were widowed, 6% were divorced or separated, and 14% had never married), and about 63% had no living children (National Center for Health Statistics, May 14, 1987). Those who have children have fewer children, older children, and children who are more geographically distant than those of the noninstitutionalized (Brody, 1981).

It is often assumed that nursing home placement signals relief of caregiver strain. Contrary to popular belief, the family does not cease its supportive activities when the older person enters an institution (Brody, 1981). Nor do family strains disappear, though they may derive from different factors. Many clinical reports describe the continuation of family concern, interest, and contacts with institutionalized older people. Family members talk to nursing home personnel about the older person, worry, feel guilty at having placed the patient (no matter how clearly the harsh realities had dictated that placement), are sad at seeing the older person's continuing decline, and experience depression and anxiety about their own aging. They may be upset about the quality of care or staff attitudes, but are often in a bind—afraid to complain because they fear retaliation on the patient. When the patient has Alzheimer's disease, that fear is intensified because the older person is relatively helpless, cannot communicate her needs to staff, and cannot report any negative treatment she may receive.

George's study of caregivers of Alzheimer's patients found that there were no significant differences in mental health, stress symptoms, and physical health between caregivers whose patients resided in long-term care facilities and those caregivers whose patients actually lived in their caregivers' households. When the same families were followed up a year later (George, 1984b), caregivers who had placed the patient in a nursing home during the previous year were more likely to be taking psychotropic drugs than were those who cared for their patients in the community or whose patients had died. Those who had placed their patients equaled those who were caring for the patients in their own homes in reporting stress symptoms and in low levels of life-satisfaction and emotional well-being. A large study of the adult children of nursing home residents also documented the strains of having an institutionalized parent. As with community studies, daughters experienced more mental health and emotional problems than sons (Brody, Dempsey, & Pruchno, 1990).

There is little research specific to the family relationships of institutionalized older people with Alzheimer's disease. One set of findings from a treatment project for cognitively impaired elderly women who lived in a nursing home indicated that such relationships remain important to both the older people and their family members. The elderly women's emotional investment in their families had risen in relative importance between their middle years and old age (Kleban, Brody, & Lawton, 1971), perhaps because other sources of emotional supplies had become depleted. Moreover, the quality of the relationships of the elderly people with their families improved in response to counseling intervention (Brody, Kleban, Lawton, & Silverman, 1971). The degree of the older person's cognitive impairment affected family visiting in that visits to the more deeply impaired institutional residents were as frequent as to those with milder impairment, but were shorter and less enjoyable to the family member. Most of the relatives reported worrying about the old person and discussing her frequently with other family members (Moss & Kurland, 1979).

Caregiving as a Social Problem

The urgency of finding ways to support caregiving families and mitigate their burdens is underlined by demographic and social trends that call into question the capacity of the family to continue to be the source of care to the same extent as in the past and at present. The birthrate continues to fall and to alter the ratio of potential care providers to care recipients. Middle-aged daughters who provide the bulk of care have been entering the work force at a very rapid rate; about 60% of parent-caring women are in the labor force (Stone et al., 1987). Increasing mobility results in geographic distance between elderly parents and adult children. The impact of rising divorce and remarriage rates on provision of care to the elderly is not known. Other complicating trends are the increase in childless couples and the later ages at which women are marrying and having a first child.

In that context, a report by the Office of Technical Assistance (OTA) points out that

> The increasing number of patients with dementia often cannot get medical, mental health, and social services from sources outside their family. Social service programs are typically intended for target populations, and those with dementia may not qualify. Many programs for the aged often exclude the mentally impaired and are not helpful to those with dementia. Programs that address social rather than medical needs usually are not covered by government health programs or standard health insurance. And the kind of coordination between medical and social services necessary for patients with dementia is unavailable in most public or private systems.
>
> An increasing number of dementia patients and their families are finding the enormous burden of care unbearable. These patients and families seek either outside assistance or nursing home placement. Medicare, Medicaid and private insurance are often inadequate, because:
>
> - Most private insurance does not cover long-term care.
> - Federal and State coverage of long-term care is being reduced as part of the effort to contain public health costs.
> - Medicare reimbursement is limited to short-term, acute-care home and nursing home coverage, yet most patients with dementia need primarily personal care, supervision, and care that lasts for years.
> - Medicaid pays the cost of institutional care only for the

indigent, and the range and quality of care vary widely from State to State and within States. To qualify for Medicaid, many patients with dementia and their families must impoverish themselves by "spending down" to eligibility. (U.S. Congress, OTA, 1987)

RESPITE CARE IN THE UNITED STATES

Respite care has emerged as the greatest unmet need expressed by caregivers, a finding that is consistent in recent research studies (Crossman, London, & Barry, 1981; Danis, 1978; Horowitz & Dobrof, 1982; Whitfield, 1981; Zimmer & Sainer, 1978). Despite the acknowledged need for that service, however, when the Philadelphia Geriatric Center (PGC) wrote a proposal for a respite service project in 1983 there were virtually no organized programs using a variety of kinds of respite service or focusing exclusively on families with Alzheimer's patients. Since then, projects of many types have proliferated.

Formal respite care in the United States was originally developed in the 1960s to serve families of developmentally disabled and retarded children who were being discharged from state facilities as part of the deinstitutionalization movement. Respite service for families of the aged is a very recent development and is one of a variety of efforts that aim to relieve caregivers' strains, thereby postponing or preventing nursing home placement. Such programs are more common in European countries, particularly the United Kingdom, where they have been in existence for a quarter of a century. For example, temporary admissions to long-stay institutions or separate facilities often takes place in parts of the United Kingdom where it is thought that the security of knowing such admissions are possible enables families to go on giving care (Gibson, 1982). Such admissions may be to hospitals, homes under voluntary auspices, or foster homes. Other countries, too, have been experimenting with institutional and community service models. An early program, beginning in 1964 at the Cowley Road Hospital in the United Kingdom offered a form of respite known as the "floating bed" program—that is, periodic planned admissions of patients. One report on that program (Robertson, Griffiths, & Cosin, 1977) concerned 50 severely disabled older people randomly selected from participants in the program. The old people received 3-day/2-night readmissions biweekly, plus intermittent longer admissions. The families rated the program as "useful" or "very useful."

In this country, some form of respite care is occasionally available through programs designed for other purposes or is embedded in more comprehensive service programs. For example, hospice programs for dying patients usually include some institutional respite care as one component of their services, day care and day hospitals have the effect of relieving caregivers and some hospitals have recently begun to market their beds for "vacation stays" for the same purpose. There is no regular public or private funding for consistent support of respite care, however. Rather, there are episodic and discontinuous efforts to provide respite of various types through privately financed demonstration grants, Medicaid waivers and other funding mechanisms (e.g., state revenues, Title XX, Title XIX, and Older American Act funds). Almost invariably, such programs are viewed as methods of postponing or avoiding institutionalization by encouraging family support.

Despite the stirrings of interest and action, a 1982 summary paper by the Center for the Study of Social Policy (Meltzer, 1982, p. 10) pointed out that there was "very little research and practice knowledge to guide program development" in respite care. The various state attempts have been characterized by variability in definitions of respite care, eligibility criteria (income, level of care needed), eligible providers, financing, and so on. For example, among the various requirements are: the disabled person must meet medical criteria for skilled nursing care; the person must be developmentally disabled; no other relative can be available to provide respite to the caregiver; the respite care must be provided to prevent institutionalization; or the patient's income must be at or below the Medicaid eligibility level. The Meltzer report concluded that there was "not a lot of evaluative knowledge about the extent of need, the costs of providing respite care, the best ways of organizing, financing and providing access to care, and the impact of offering respite care as a support for family caregiving" (p. 25).

A similar conclusion was drawn by another 1982 summary report:

> Little research has been done to examine the effectiveness of these various options. Evaluation of service programs to look at demand, costs, and outcomes would be useful for those in the process of developing a respite care policy or program. Research is needed to determine how families care for their aged dependent and the type of supports that would provide the most help at the least cost. It would be useful to look at the benefits of respite care programs in terms of the caregivers' and dependents' psychological and physical well-being and their contribution to family support of the elderly, as well as the most cost efficient way of providing such services. The variety of needs and circumstances that are experienced by families suggests that a wide range of services and facilities and a variety of funding sources may be an appropriate approach to the development of respite care services. (Yocom, 1982, p. 14)

During the last several years, respite care service programs have proliferated nationally. Although there is no uniform definition of respite, it is generally defined as any service or group of services designed to provide caregivers with temporary or short-term relief away from the disabled person. These programs are diverse, varying from one another in refinements of the definition of respite, target population(s), auspices, funding streams, types and amounts of respite offered, and service models. In some programs, for example, "temporary" can refer to substitute care while the caregiver works, while in others, working caregivers are excluded. Some programs exclude emergency care while others include it, and some programs offer only emergency, temporary care (Texas Department of Human Resources, 1982). In some programs, respite care is clearly differentiated from long term-care (Mosley, 1983). Others do not make such a clear differentiation, but the limited amounts of services available do not satisfy needs for long-term care. Definition and program purpose are often linked;

programs with Medicaid funding combine the goal of providing caregiver relief with the goal of reducing institutional care.

Characteristics of Respite Clients

The target populations vary significantly from program to program. A few programs serve only caregivers of Alzheimer's patients (Gold, 1986; Spence & Miller, 1985/86; Seltzer, Fabiszewaski, Brown, & Lyon, 1985), while some serve the general population of chronically disabled people, including children (California Department of Mental Health, 1987; Connecticut Department of Health Services, 1983; Wisconsin Department of Health and Social Services, 1983; Yocum, 1982). Most, however, target an older population with physical and mental disabilities in which Alzheimer's patients constitute a substantial number of those served (Dunn, 1986; Munson, 1983; Rowland, 1985). But many programs exclude those whose severe disabilities are beyond the capabilities of staff. In addition to age and disability criteria, project recipients may also need to meet other criteria such as eligibility for skilled or intermediate nursing home care (Palmer, 1981), VA status (Ellis & Wilson, 1983) or disabled spouse status (Crossman et al., 1981).

Sponsorship of Programs

Respite programs are operated by a variety of agencies and organizations such as government agencies, volunteer organizations, and home health care agencies. The majority of programs operate with mixed streams of funding. Funding can be through government funds, foundations (Crozier, 1982; Spence & Miller, 1985/86), religious institutions (Adult Services, 1984; Hornbaker, 1983; National Council of Catholic Women, 1983), and caregiver/family resources. Family cost sharing often is a key requirement and may vary from flexible, modest family donations (Gold, 1986) to set fees and sliding-scale formulae (Hevern, 1985; Wisconsin Department of Health and Social Services, 1983). Middle- and upper-income families may be excluded from programs targeted to those with low incomes (Dixon-Bemis, 1986).

Funding

There is a growing trend for government resources to fund respite programs. Such government funding is most often through AOA Title III of the Older Americans Act and/or Title XX of the Social Security Act (Dunn, 1986; Hornbaker, 1983; Munson, 1983), Medicaid (Connecticut Department of Health Services, 1983; Palmer, 1981; Rowland, 1985), and Medicare waivers (Montgomery, 1988). By 1985, 15 states had some mention of respite in legislation; allocations were generally small, however, and often only for time-limited demonstrations (see Stone, 1986 for review). When program funding includes Medicaid, it is likely that family income is an eligibility criterion. In at least two government-financed projects, different models were tested in demonstrations (Montgomery, 1988; Rabbit, 1986).

Respite Service Organization

Respite programs have varied types of relationships with the actual providers of the respite service. Some programs employ the staff and/or own the facilities that are used for actual respite such as day-care centers, corps of in-home respite staff, and institutional facilities (Ellis & Wilson, 1983). Other programs have formal subcontractual relationships with providers (Munson, 1983) and are responsible for funding, setting standards, and monitoring and evaluating service provision.

Recognizing the shortage of trained respite-provider staff, some programs have designed special training programs (Hornbaker, 1983; Wiskovsky, 1986). Another staffing option is the use of volunteers, most often with professionals doing the recruitment, training, and supervision (Adult Services, 1984; Evans, 1985; McGuane, 1989). Still another variation is the cooperative model (U.S. Department of Health and Human Services, 1986; Vintage, Inc., 1985)—that is, a care exchange, with families taking turns providing care to each other's elders. Care rendered is paid for by care to be delivered, and there is no exchange of money.

Types of Respite Care

Types of respite and the amounts available also vary. *In-home respite* refers to companions, homemakers, volunteers, and home-health care aides who come into the caregiver's home. In a few programs, the disabled person is taken to the home of the respite worker (U.S. Department of Health and Human Services, 1986; Vintage, Inc., 1985). *Day care* refers to attendance at day centers ranging from small socialization/sitter programs (National Council of Catholic Women, 1983) to large, professionally staffed programs with multiple types of services in addition to respite. *Overnight, out-of-home respite* refers to short-term stays in nursing homes, hospitals, and other congregate settings such as foster homes and group homes (Crossman, et al., 1981; Hildebrandt, 1983; Russell, 1983; Texas Department of Human Resources, 1982; Wisconsin Department of Health and Social Services, 1983). Some programs offer only one type of respite, usually in-home (Adult Services, 1984; Crozier, 1982; Evans, 1985; Mosley, 1983; National Council of Catholic Women, 1983; Vintage, Inc., 1985; Wiskovsky, 1986; Yocum, 1982), while others offer options (Connecticut Department of Health Services, 1983; Crossman, et al., 1981; Hevern, 1985; Munson, 1983; Rowland, 1985; White & Ehrlich, 1988; Wisconsin Department of Health and Social Services, 1983).

Respite programs usually establish maximum hours or days of respite available to families and these also differ from program to program. Examples are: four hours weekly for in-home respite (Adult Services, 1984; Evans, 1985), one half-day weekly for day care (Gold, 1986), two weeks in an institutional setting (Seltzer et al., 1985), 164 hours of care a year (Baltimore/Central Maryland Alzheimer's Association, 1989) and a combination of respite types not in excess of 240 hours or ten days yearly (Wisconsin Department of Health and Social Services, 1983).

Caregivers often are offered more than respite service in these programs, with additional services ranging from information and referral (I&R) to comprehensive service packages. I&R, caregiver education, and support groups are the most frequently offered services, but some programs provide diagnosis, evaluation, and medical treatment (Ellis & Wilson, 1983; Seltzer et al., 1985). In other programs, respite is embedded in a constellation of long-term care (LTC) services such as case management, counseling, and home delivered meals (California Department of Mental Health, 1987; Dixon-Bemis, 1986; Munson, 1983; Palmer, 1981; Respite Care Demonstrations Projects, 1986; Rowland, 1985). Such programs are usually sponsored by government agencies and are linked to the already existing social service and aging networks.

Program Evaluation of Respite Services

During the 1980s reports began to emerge about a variety of respite projects with some form of evaluation. Many such reports were anecdotal or consisted of program descriptions. Some of the evaluations were at least partly retrospective, and rarely did an evaluation compare respite recipients with a control group. The types of respite varied, and most programs included people with all types of disabilities. Some programs embedded respite service in programs that included a wide constellation of services, while others were free-standing. Sample sizes were generally small, and most findings were based on caregivers reporting whether or not they perceived the respite as helpful or citing their levels of satisfaction with it.

The following summaries of selected projects for which some evaluation was performed is not intended to be comprehensive. Rather, the projects will illustrate the diversity of program types and the state-of-the-art.

Two reports from the Veterans Administration (VA) provide examples of studies focusing specifically on institutional respite. In one (Scharlach & Frenzel, 1986), eight beds were made available for chronically disabled veterans for up to two weeks of respite every two months, with caregivers being able to request up to 28 days once a year. Eighteen months after the program began, 99 of 150 caregivers responded to a questionnaire. Improvement in the caregivers' health was reported by 72% of them, in sleep by 55%, in relationships with the impaired person by 56%, and in the latter's health by 38%. Eighty-four percent of the caregivers said respite made it easier to continue to provide care and 70% were "very satisfied" with the service. About one-third of the respondents viewed permanent placement of the care-recipient in a nursing home as being less likely in the coming year than it would have been had respite care not been available; an almost equal proportion saw placement as being more likely.

In the other VA respite program (Seltzer et al., 1985; Seltzer et al., 1988), 36 cognitively impaired patients had a total of 61 respite admissions as part of a research/clinical program focusing on a team approach for the demented. No changes in cognitive or functional status of the patients were found for the two-week preadmission to post-test period.

An 18-month project in New York State, financed with foundation funds (Meltzer, 1982), also limited respite service to institutional care. It took place at six long-term care facilities (i.e., nursing homes) and was targeted to patients with all diagnoses who met the New York State standards for eligibility for institutional care. Most of the 134 patients in the project required skilled nursing care, and the average length of stay in the nursing homes was 18 days. Seventy-two percent of the caregivers used respite in order to take vacations or have temporary relief. The others used respite when the caregiver was ill or following a hospital stay; in these cases, it was more likely that the patient would be placed permanently in a nursing home. Families were required to pay the full cost of care ($5,000 to $12,000 annually per bed), which was high at the time because of the need to hold vacant beds. Most (78.5%) caregivers considered the service "very satisfactory" and 19.6% considered it "satisfactory." One outcome was an unexpectedly high rate of permanent institutionalization of the patients within one month of use of the respite service (12% of patients).

In a Canadian project (Dunn, MacBeath, & Robertson, 1983), respite service took place via admission to a teaching hospital. Twenty-eight families were served during a two-year period. All of the disabled people had to be eligible for institutional care; 79% of them were demented. Three types of respite were provided: (1) planned, regular, intermittent admission (89%); (2) holiday stays of up to two weeks duration once a year (8%); and (3) admission when the caregiver was hospitalized (3%). Evaluation of the program was done retrospectively by review of health records and interviews with the program social worker. At the end of the study, more than one-third of the disabled people were still living at home while half had been placed in nursing homes. The authors concluded that the program had delayed nursing home admissions—a surprising conclusion in view of the very high rate of such admissions.

Miller, Gulle, & McCue, (1986) reported a respite program in which 16 patients received residential respite in an apartment and six in a nursing home. The frail elderly patients included some with Alzheimer's disease. For residential and nursing home respite the per diem cost was $60 and $120, respectively, with financial assistance available if income and residency requirements could not be met. The findings were derived from a questionnaire completed by the program social workers who had questioned other staff. Seven caregivers were judged to be "enthusiastic" about the program, four to be "satisfied," four to be dissatisfied, and three to be more open to long-term care placement.

A demonstration in which several types of respite care were combined was the Wives' Respite Project (Crossman et al., 1981). Services included home care, over-night respite in a six-bed residential facility, and education. A small program in Marin County, California, it provided respite care to wives of disabled husbands but was not available to husbands of disabled women or to other caregiving relatives such as adult children. The disabled husbands included the physically disabled as well as those with mental impairments. The program was offered only to members of a wives' support group (average attendance was 10–15 wives per week). There was no formal research evaluation of this program, though the report states that a "client satisfaction survey" took place with the wives reporting that it was successful in relieving their burdens. The women expressed "deep gratitude" for being able to get out of the house and for the peace, quiet, and rest they enjoyed.

An example of a day-care program for Alzheimer's patients is the Harbor Area Adult Day Care Center in Costa Mesa, California. Typically, this center has the goal of combining respite for caregivers with a meaningful experience for an average daily census of 20 care-recipients. Day care is combined with counseling, referrals, and monthly support meetings for the caregivers. Though there has been no formal evaluation, a report (Sands & Suzuki, 1983) stated that most of its clients said they otherwise would have to use 24-hour care (i.e., in a nursing home), and that they received relief, insight, and emotional support as a result of the program. Funding came from clients (47%) and donations (43%), and the cost at the time was $23.35 per day.

Rather than being offered as a discrete service, a multi service respite program for low-income persons in Pima County, Arizona, is a component of an array of many programs comprising the county's long-term care system (Dixon-Bemis, 1986). It includes in-home, day care, and nursing home respite and is designed not only to relieve the caregiver for a period of time but also to relieve her of some caregiving tasks. Embedding respite in a system of other services—including strong case management—permits program flexibility and the accommodation of different levels and types of needs. For example, the program provides three types of day care (for physically impaired elderly, Alzheimer's patients, and young disabled adults). Most clients are served by the in-home programs, however; about 1600 people are served on any given day of whom 75% receive services that include a respite component. Dixon-Bemis' description (1986) of this conceptually sophisticated program notes some issues and pitfalls. Limited resources compel difficult decisions such as whether the service should be aimed at the caregiver or the impaired person (e.g., relief for the caregiver or a bath for the impaired person?). Other dilemmas are whether the resources should be used for preventive or maintenance care, whether resources should be allocated to one high-need situation versus distribution of that amount of service to five or six families, and the relatively high cost of in-home respite vis-á-vis institutional care. This report, too, notes the lack of caregiver education about and acceptance of the respite concept.

A small program staffed by volunteers is being demonstrated at three sites in New York City (two churches and a synagogue) (Quinn & Crabtree, 1987). Financed by the Brookdale Foundation, Alzheimer's patients who are not severely impaired are offered socialization and activities while their caregivers have respite. Caregivers are also referred elsewhere for services beyond the scope of the program. Volunteers staff the programs under the leadership of a professional. No data are available, but anecdotal reports indicate beneficial effects for caregivers and care recipients. Based on experience with the demonstration, a guide has been written for communities wishing to start similar programs (Quinn & Crabtree, 1987).

An ambitious research and demonstration project at the University of Washington—The Family Support Project—tested five different models of family support programs to over 541 caregiving families who were assigned to one of the experimental models or to a control group (Montgomery, 1988). In one model, eight hours of volunteer respite per month were provided through a local home health agency. In another, paid respite services were provided through Medicare waivers, with families able to choose the provider (nursing home, home-health agency and/or adult day care center) and the duration of the care. Information is available about the volunteer component (Montgomery, 1986; Montgomery & Borgatta, 1985), which served 306 families, and about a comparison between the control group and two of the experimental service models that included respite care (Montgomery, 1988).

In the volunteer program, the characteristics of the impaired older people were similar to those of nursing home residents (average age of 81, almost one-half with serious problems due to "mental impairment"). Those being cared for by spouses were younger, but more impaired functionally than those being cared for by adult children. Most caregivers were female (79%), and were predominantly either a child (57%) or a spouse (37%). Caregivers' median age was 62 (58 for children and 71 for spouses); most were married and about one-third were employed. Caregivers spent a mean of 36 hours weekly in caregiving and, as in other studies, there was minimal use of formal services. Using a "controlled experimental design," it was found that the objective burden of spouse caregivers who received the volunteer respite was significantly lower than that of spouses who were not eligible for the service.

Again it was found that recruiting participants and encouraging use of respite was a problem; typically requests were made after the situation had reached crisis proportions. Recruitment of volunteers willing to provide individual services for an extended time also was extremely difficult. The disabled elderly clients required a level of care beyond the capacities of the volunteers.

Montgomery and Prothero (1986) have edited a book on respite that includes case material, their initial findings from the project, and several chapters authored by people operating other respite projects. Rabbit (1986) describes the large respite demonstration project initiated by New York State, which also aimed to test different models. The state provided funds for administration, but not for the respite service per se. The definition of respite included the phrase "infrequent and temporary substitute care." Seven sites were selected to demonstrate various approaches. Only a preliminary evaluation is available as yet, which describes the projects and the various kinds of difficulties they have encountered operationally. For example, in the Allentown Community Center project in Buffalo, in-home respite, supportive skill-building, and health maintenance opportunities to caregivers are provided by trained peer paraprofessionals and displaced caregivers. The level of care required proved to be greater than paraprofessionals could provide, however, and some of the older people were more appropriate for placement in a long-term care facility.

Problems encountered by other models in the New York State project included unsuitable site selection, cost barriers in a low-income area, the need for brief respite rather than for the planned 24-hour period, a shortage of nursing home beds for institutional respite, and the need to mount public information programs to educate and recruit caregivers. Rabbit's interim report (1986) states experience with the 650 families who have been served indicates that a variety of respite options are needed with different levels of care and that the typical client has a greater need for functional (ADL) assistance than for health-related services. He points out that all the projects had very slow starts compounded by the need to establish relationships among a number of different agencies and, as in so many other projects, the lack of client familiarity with respite. He concludes that no single service is sufficient and that communities need flexibility in developing services that make the best use of local resources.

The VA in Palo Alto, California has a multiservice respite program (i.e., day care, in-home, and institutional) (Ellis, 1986). In the institutional component of the program, five beds are reserved in the VA Nursing Home Care Unit with admissions scheduled at the family's request. Only confused wanderers cannot be cared for. In the year prior to Ellis' report there were 305 admissions, with the patients' levels of disability being much more severe than anticipated. No data are available as yet from studies of the program, but it has been very successful operationally (full bed occupancy), with clients (caregivers *and* patients) expressing satisfaction and looking forward to admissions. Again, as in many other reports, the initial reluctance of clients to use the service is noted.

Respite was one of the services in a comprehensive program for brain-damaged adults (most of whom had dementia) (California Department of Mental Health, 1987). It was defined as up to 72 hours of emergency care. Respite was authorized in eight of the 1,145 cases screened at intake, but only four actually used it, of whom three recipients evaluated the service favorably on a questionnaire.

The state of Washington mounted an ambitious program in which 619 families were served in three demonstrations (Respite Care Demonstration Project, Olympia, WA, 1986). Seventy-one percent of the patients were described as being disoriented or having memory loss, with most being very disabled. Three-fifths of them were 75 years of age or over. The caregivers' mean age was 65 and most were wives of the patients; two-thirds of them had their own health problems and 76% suffered stress effects. The total of 61,000 hours of respite over a 16-months period cost $632 per family, which the authors of the report point out is far less than the cost of nursing home care. Short periods of respite (up to eight hours at a time) were preferred. The report recommends offering 576 hours of respite annually and requiring that caregivers participate in the costs.

Following its surveys of the well-being of Alzheimer's caregivers who were members of support groups, Duke University mounted a respite service program (George, 1986). The program was stimulated by the finding that respite was the service most desired by the surveyed caregivers but was the least available. In two models of service, in-home respite is being provided under the sponsorship of a nursing home and by a home health agency. In a report based on the first 22 cases, caregivers report that respite care does indeed provide relief and that an added benefit is derived from the relationship between respite worker and client. Caregivers use the respite time to run errands, relax at home, and engage in leisure activities. On the minus side, they want more respite, but cost is a barrier. (Caregivers want 15–20 hours weekly, but receive an average of 8 hours since the program is capped at $32 weekly per family.) The Duke report repeats the common refrain that the demand for the service was lower than anticipated, and that caregivers find it difficult to use community services, most often failing to seek respite until the patient is far advanced in the disease process.

The Administration on Aging financed a program to test respite co-ops in Michigan—that is, projects in which caregivers would provide short-term respite to each other. One of the projects, the Elder Care Share program in Kalamazoo, is sponsored by the South Central Michigan Commission on Aging, which provides administration and guidance to the volunteers who recruit families. Though at an early phase of development, the project is having a major problem in recruiting participant families.

In a controlled study of respite that was not limited to Alzheimer's patients, almost one-third of the 189 families eligible for respite services offered through Medicare waivers failed to use any services (Montgomery, 1988). These families (unlike those in the PGC program) were applying for service and were then randomly assigned to programs consisting of various combinations of education and respite services. The majority of families chose in-home respite services for frequent periods of three hours. On the average, families spent only 63% of their allotted funds. Respite appeared to delay nursing home placement among families with adult children as caregivers but encouraged placement when spouses were the primary caregivers. Although no overall effect on subjective burden was observed, for the families whose older member remained in the community for the full treatment year, a significant reduction in burden was measured for respite recipients but not for members of the control group.

The most recent major effort is sponsored by the Robert Wood Johnson Foundation. Twenty-two demonstration sites were selected from the 283 that responded to the Foundation's request for proposals. Begun in 1988, this four-year project will test the effectiveness of a variety of locally-determined respite packages. Three are operated directly by Alzheimer's Association chapters, 9 are affiliated with local chapters, and 10 are based in existing agencies. Another contrast is between the free-standing respite services (the 12 related to the Association) and the multiservice agency-based respite programs.

The Health Care Financing Administration, in response to a congressional mandate in the Omnibus Budget Reconciliation Act of 1986, has launched its Medicare Alzheimer's Disease Demonstration Project. The demonstration component located in several national sites will provide a rich array of services, including respite options to Medicare beneficiaries with Alzheimer's disease and their families. The project's research evaluation component will determine the effectiveness, cost, and impact on health status and functioning of providing comprehensive services to Medicare recipients and their families. This three-year project is currently in its planning stage.

Another multi-site demonstration program has been established by the Brookdale Foundation, using the basic Brookdale model (Quinn & Crabtree, 1987), but encouraging local variations among the nine sites.

CONCLUSION

Several themes recur in descriptions of respite programs. First, there are problems in getting enough respite to fill the needs due to fiscal limitations. Second, respite is the most wished for but least available service. Third, most caregivers are not familiar with the concept of respite and do not avail themselves of the service until they are at an end-point of stress. Fourth, families are often reluctant to use respite and when they do so, use it modestly.

The PGC project to be described in the next chapter is unique in that no other respite program focusing on caregivers of Alzheimer's victims has been evaluated by means of a controlled multifaceted research design. Nor has any other program focusing on the needs of such caregivers organized a constellation of as many different types of respite services, packaged flexibly to meet each family's particular and changing needs. Finally, the PGC program is the only one of which we are aware in which respondents volunteered to participate in a research study and were assigned to experimental or control groups after the initial assessment. This made it possible to estimate service yield for a given population more accurately.

The Experimental Family Respite Care Service Program

2

In the demonstration program, respite services were offered to those caregivers designated as members of the experimental (intervention) group. This chapter will focus on that program and those who participated in it. The services and procedures will be described—both the respite services and the context of services designed to facilitate and enable use of respite. Case excerpts will illustrate situations in which caregivers were enabled to avail themselves of respite, situations in which caregivers refused respite, and reasons for such refusal.

THE VARIETIES OF RESPITE CARE

The respite program (Family Respite Care Service Program [FRCP]) carried out by the PGC was designed to support the relatives who had the major responsibility for the care of the Alzheimer's patients. Family situations were expected to be diverse in many ways. For example, the primary caregivers could be spouses, adult children, or other relatives. Socioeconomic status, living arrangements, work status, ethnicity, preferences, and other family characteristics also were expected to vary. In order to meet the different needs of such different families, a variety of services were planned that could be mobilized in individualized packages tailored to the needs of each family. It was intended that the care provided to the Alzheimer's patients would be of high quality and tailored to their unique needs not only in terms of the services, but also for special understanding and management (for example, preparing them for services and orienting them to new people and new places).

The Respite Services

Respite care was defined for purposes of the program as *"any service or group of services designed to provide temporary periods of relief and/or rest for caregivers away from the patient."* This inclusive definition meant that the program's services could:

- be provided by informal sources (family or friends) or formal sources (government, social/health agencies, or independent paid workers);
- be subsidized by the project, government or nonprofit organizations, or paid for from the patient's or family's own resources;
- take place *in the home* of the patient/family or *out of the home* (for example, in a day care program or in a facility such as a nursing home or other institution);
- be planned in advance for *special purposes* (such as short family vacations, caregivers' attendance at events such as weddings or medical/dental appointments) or for *routine periodic relief* (e.g., a free afternoon or evening weekly);
- respond to unexpected circumstances, providing the caregiver with the security of knowing back-up was available for emergencies such as illness of the caregiver or caregiver's spouse;
- be provided to caregivers who had not already been using respite services or to supplement those already being used by families.

Only needed services not otherwise available were created by the project; those already in existence at the PGC or at other community agencies would be used but would not be duplicated. The Foundation grant made purchase of services possible and they were available in sufficient quantity. The program was open to people of all socioeconomic and ethnic backgrounds and there were no financial eligibility criteria.

It should be remembered that the caregivers in the program had not requested respite service or responded to an announcement that such services were available. Rather, they had volunteered to participate in a research study, had received a baseline assessment, and only then were assigned randomly to the control (no-service) and respite service groups.

The program made not only the respite services but also certain core services available to the participants.

The *respite services* offered were of several types:

1. *Out-of-home respite care—Institutional respite.* Beds were made available in the nursing home and in the hospital of the Philadelphia Geriatric Center. (One section of the PGC skilled nursing facility was designed specifically for people with Alzheimer's disease.) These beds were used for both *emergency* respite care (e.g., illness of caregiver or a member of caregiver's family) and *planned* respite (e.g., for a caregiver's short vacation or weekend relaxation or simply to meet her need for a rest).

2. *Out-of-home respite care—Day care.* Day care was made available for varying amounts of time (that is, for one to five days weekly) in the PGC's Day Center or in other day centers in the city (if appropriate and available). (At the outset of the project, there were about 10 day care centers in the Philadelphia area.)

3. *In-home respite care.* This type of care took place in the home in which the Alzheimer's patient lived. It was provided by an appropriate nonprofessional whose services were purchased from another agency and who worked under supervision. Depending on the caregiver's need, the in-home care was regular (e.g., a one-half day weekly) or occasional (on request) and took place during the day, in the evening, or for a weekend. The qualifications of the particular surrogate caregiver provided by the project depended on the individ-

ual situation. A patient who also was physically ill or severely impaired functionally, for example, required a more highly skilled worker than the patient whose problem was solely confusion requiring round-the-clock supervision.

4. *Care-sharing.* Research indicates that in most cases, the burden of care is borne primarily by one person in the family—the spouse when one exists, an adult child or child-in-law, or occasionally a sibling who is elderly herself. In appropriate situations, therefore, other members of the families were encouraged to provide some respite care. The family situation was explored with the utmost delicacy and skill and the suggestion made only to selected families so as not to upset the family's balance of relationships.

Another form of care-sharing was also explored—specifically, the possibility that caregivers from different families might exchange relief with each other.

PLANNING AND PROCEDURES

Preliminary Planning

As a basis for planning for respite care, caregivers in the program were asked what services they were currently using, their past use of respite, and the kind of respite services they would like to have. They were given an explanation of how the latter services could be used and a brochure describing those different uses. The interviewer explained how she would work during the next year as a case manager, collaborating with the caregiver to identify formal and informal respite service and facilitate their use. When indicated, specific respite options were explored in preparation for a follow-up meeting the following week at which concrete plans would be made.

The interviewer's observations of the caregiver and the latter's environment were recorded, and a file was created to record pertinent information and case activity. Each caregiver received a letter of appreciation and $25 for completing the initial home interview.

Follow-up and Monitoring

Planning continued during the follow-up contacts. A staff member worked as an ongoing facilitator with each caregiver to identify respite care needs and resources, to develop an individualized plan, to determine the method of payment for the service, and to implement the plan and modify it as the needs changed.

If a participant wanted respite service but hesitated to use it because of financial constraints, the case manager explained the financial subsidies available from the project. The caregiver was asked how much the family could afford to pay, and the remaining costs were subsidized based on the incomes of both the impaired person and caregiver, the appropriateness of respite service (i.e., temporary relief from caregiving rather than a total long-term care program), and the limits of the program budget. An agreement, signed by both caregiver and worker and reviewed periodically, detailed the type of respite service and the amount to be paid by the family. Because the source of payment for respite is a social policy issue and is often problematic for program planners, the procedure used will be elaborated here.

Payment for the Experimental Respite Services

Families' attitudes towards money can prevent use of vitally needed respite. Determination of the manner in which each family's respite service was to be financed was one of the most difficult tasks of the initial stages of the project. While the per diem and hourly costs of the various services were known, there was absolutely no information about how much service might be needed and used. The demonstration grant included a fixed amount of funds with which to subsidize service. The policy of the project, however, was that families participate in paying if they could afford to do so. But how was that amount to be determined? An arbitrary sliding scale could be too liberal or too harsh and families had different needs in other areas of their lives. Moreover, because one of the project aims was to estimate the potential cost of respite to the community, it was considered undesirable to inhibit service use artificially.

Resolving the dilemma with respect to family cost-sharing was facilitated by exploring the payment issue tentatively with the first 10 or 15 families entering the program. It soon became apparent that their demands for service were modest and that they preferred to participate in payment. The decision was made, therefore, to cap the amount of subsidizing funds that would usually be made available at $1,000 per family for the service year. The amount was arrived at by the practical expedient of dividing the amount of money available in the grant by the number of families we expected to serve. It was recognized, however, that some families might need in excess of $1,000 and the cap was therefore flexible in order to respond to special needs. When it appeared that a particular family needed more than that amount, the situation was discussed with and cleared by the project director. This system proved to be controllable and equitable.

Nevertheless, the financial cost of caring for the impaired family members was a major concern of the caregivers. Despite the offer of the subsidy, families who felt respite was needed often told staff that cost was a major obstacle to use or greater use of service. This was one of the reasons that families sometimes delayed using respite until they "really needed it," first extending themselves to the point of mental and physical exhaustion.

Determination of what a family's contributions should be was a delicate matter. Before using the financial subsidy, it was necessary to evaluate the family's capacity to contribute. Most families initiated the subject of costs themselves, prefacing their request for service with the assertion that they wanted to contribute. And they did so. Some contributed nominal amounts, such as $1.00 for each respite episode. Others, with greater financial means, paid three-fourths of the costs. There is consensus among project staff that the vast majority of caregivers were more than receptive to paying whatever they could afford. In fact, the workers suspected at times that families were paying more than they could comfortably manage.

> An extremely poor but proud caregiver requested institutional respite for her severely impaired husband when she required surgery. She insisted on paying half the costs (she paid with small bills) and donated her handiwork to PGC's Family Fair to show her appreciation for the respite subsidy.

After the initial home assessment and follow-up, caregivers were contacted at least once every two months to monitor the situation and to carry out various case management activities that related to developing and implementing the respite plan. Clients were encouraged to call staff when they needed service or information related to their caregiving activities.

Service Termination

A one year intervention project to assist caregivers with needs that may have existed for as long as ten years must allow sufficient time for an orderly and constructive process of service termination to occur. Project staff clearly informed caregivers at the outset that service would be available only for one year. Case plans and contracts between the program and caregivers were designed to reflect that time limit. Throughout the project year, every effort was made to educate caregivers about existing community services and to link them to services under other auspices that they could continue to use after the termination of the experimental program.

Approximately two months before the end of the project, participants were reminded that the program would be ending. Social workers and caregivers discussed ongoing or anticipated needs and resources that might be available. Literature on a separate service for community residents, the PGC's Counseling for Caregivers (CFC) Program, was given to them and those who wished were contacted by that program. When indicated, a counseling service social worker accompanied the project social worker for the final visit to the caregiver's home to ensure continuity of service. (Approximately 80 caregivers were contacted by the counseling service as they ended their year with the project.)

COMPONENTS OF THE RESPITE SERVICE

Regardless of the type(s) of respite used, the program was guided by an overall philosophy and contained certain common elements. The services included:

1. *Information and referral (I&R)* by a project staff member (social worker or nurse). The staff person was responsible for assisting each family to design its individual respite program, linking the various services to each other, monitoring the situation throughout the service period, and modifying the service package as dictated by the changing needs of the family.

2. *Transportation* (if needed). Because lack of transportation to bring a disabled older person to the site of service delivery (e.g., to a day-care program) can be a major barrier to service utilization, one of the PGC hydraulic lift vans was used when other modes of transportation were not available.

It was accepted as a given that the sheer existence of any service does not insure its use; rather, it must be embedded in a counseling process and linked to a constellation of other services. To accomplish its goal, therefore, the respite model included those other services that were deemed to be essential to appropriate utilization of the respite—specifically, assessment, education, case management, and counseling.

Most caregivers in the respite program proved to require those services to enable them to use respite and to do so effectively. At the beginning of their participation, they had different levels of knowledge and were at different stages of readiness to use the service.

Assessment, education, case management, and counseling are by no means mutually exclusive, of course, but often overlap and blend one with the others. In reading the description of those four services, therefore, it is important to keep in mind that they do not fall into discrete categories. With the exception of the standardized research assessment protocol administered during the first contact, the timing, types, and amounts of the various services were dictated by each family's unique set of needs as determined by their expressed needs and good clinical practice. During the one-year service period, detailed records were kept noting the amounts of time staff spent in these various service activities. To some extent, the notations were arbitrary as each activity contains elements of the others. The time estimates below, therefore, only approximate the allocation of worker time. Similarly, the definitions of services depict the range of activities though they cannot always be teased apart completely.

Assessment

A key service offered to all project families was a broad-based in-home assessment on which subsequent intervention was predicted. The assessment had two major components: the research instrument, and the clinical information and observations obtained in the initial contacts between the case manager (social worker)* and the family. The focus of both was primarily on the caregiver: her health, patterns of socialization and recreation, financial status, psychological status, environment, the family support and social service resources available to her, and her perceived burden and problems. Information was also gathered about the impaired person including, for example, the duration of the illness, health status, behavioral symptoms, and functional capacities.

The data and the worker's judgments about the family's problems and strengths formed the basis of the initial case plan. When respite was refused initially, periodic contact was

*"Case manager" and "worker" as used in this report refer to the respite workers who were (with one exception) professional social workers. The exception was a registered nurse.

maintained to identify ways in which staff could be helpful, to strengthen and maintain the worker/caregiver relationship, and to lay the groundwork for modifying the plan in accordance with any changes over time that occurred in the needs of the caregiver and patient. The processes of informal assessment and case planning, therefore, were ongoing; each family was contacted at two month intervals and more frequently as indicated.

The formal assessment served several other purposes in addition to being the basic research instrument.

First, because the assessment protocol covered all relevant areas systematically, caregivers were helped to identify problem areas and concerns that might otherwise have been overlooked. Such coverage of specific issues also enabled them to recognize ways in which they had coped successfully with difficult situations. In answering specific questions about patient behaviors and how they had been managed, for example, many respondents realized that they had coped quite effectively with difficult behaviors.

Second, the strains experienced by caregivers may have led them to subjective and confusing perceptions of situations and problems. Because the assessment questions were anchored in the specifics of function, caregivers were helped to view their situations more objectively and to differentiate problems.

Third, by helping caregivers to reframe overwhelming feelings and to identify specific problems that were amenable to solution, assessment served as the initial step toward ameliorating or resolving those problems.

Fourth, the assessment process set the stage for a sharp focus on the caregiver's needs. A first step for a significant number of them was to recognize that they too had needs that were legitimate and that differed from those of the patients.

Finally, a most significant value of the assessment process was that it was key to establishing a helping relationship between worker and caregiver.

Determination of whether respite service was appropriate was a crucial element of the assessment process and the development of a care plan. The project viewed respite not as a substitute for a comprehensive long-term care plan, but as a potential component of such a plan. Some caregivers did indeed need comprehensive planning for long-term care. There were times, however, when the views of the project staff and the caregiver did not mesh with another agency's criteria for respite or long-term care services. In a few cases, for example, project staff judged that long-term care services were needed, while another agency viewed the situation as requiring only respite services. Such differences in perspective may be due to the fact that long-term care agencies almost invariably focus on the needs of the impaired person, principally those who live alone. As a result, services are often denied when a caregiver is present and available. Indeed, many long-term care systems are so hampered by lack of funding that they are unable to provide care even for desperately needy older persons who live alone.

Caregiver Education

The caregivers were educated about respite care and about dementia, and were prepared for changes that might occur in the future.

Education About Respite Care

About two-thirds of FRCP caregivers required and received educational services to familiarize them with the concept of respite. Education included familiarizing them with the meaning and purposes of respite. A potential obstacle in using such service is that the concept is new to many caregivers. Most families in the program did not know what respite service was and initially did not view it as a real alternative that was applicable to their own situations. Very few understood respite as a means of preventing or mitigating their ongoing burdens and strains. Rather, most thought of it as a service to be used only when they could no longer manage at all.

Initially, almost all participants required multiple explanations about respite and how it could apply to their own unique set of circumstances. For some, repeated explanations continued throughout the project year. Families who did not grasp the concept even after multiple explanations were given a brochure with definitions and descriptions of respite options. There were, of course, some exceptions. A small group of families readily recognized their need for respite and did not require extensive explanations.

Education About Dementia

Because most of the patients had not received a complete diagnostic evaluation, there were gaps in caregivers' information about the symptoms of the disease, its progression, and ways of coping with behaviors. It was not uncommon for them to attribute disease symptoms to the victim's personality: "He just does that to annoy me," or "If only she would pay attention, she wouldn't be so forgetful." Information was provided about dementia, its manifestations and ways of coping with different patient behaviors, and about changes that might occur in the future. When incontinence was a problem, for example, toileting every two hours might be suggested. Families were told how to distract patients who persisted in a potentially harmful activity such as trying to get out of the house. Some caregivers were particularly distressed because they attributed the patient's crying, pacing, and flattened affect to unhappiness and depression. Such matters were discussed with the family, books and articles were recommended, and referrals were made to the Alzheimer's Association. This educational process helped participants to respond to upsetting patient behaviors in more constructive ways.

Preparation for Change

Caregivers were sometimes unaware that they might need help and support from others in the future and some were unaware of the existence of community resources. A resource guide developed by the project staff was given to them after the initial assessment and again one year later at the end of the service program. The need for long-range planning was emphasized because of the inevitable changes that would occur in the patient's condition and functioning. This approach seemed to mitigate caregivers' stress not only because it helped to prepare them for changes but also because they were able to develop a plan to deal with such potential changes, rather than facing an unknown and frightening future. The following case excerpt illustrates such education:

> An elderly caregiver who was managing his wife's care quite well with help from their daughters was concerned about the future. Would his wife's condition deteriorate? What would happen to her if he became ill? With the social worker's encouragement, he brought his family together for a meeting. The social worker and the family discussed respite and long-term care options. Information about the disease's progression was shared with the family and they were given reading materials about Alzheimer's disease and resource information. As a result of this meeting, the family explored and located in-home service agencies, nursing home respite facilities and two long-term care nursing home facilities in case the need arose. Although the family did not use respite during the project year, the caregiver felt relieved and more secure because he was prepared for the future.

Case Management

Case management—that is, information and referral, connecting families to needed services provided by community agencies and monitoring the situation over time—was a major component of the service model. About half of the participants in the program were provided with help to link them to other service agencies and resources. About three times more service time was spent in case management than in education or counseling.

The amounts and types of such interventions varied greatly, ranging from straightforward information and referral (I & R) to more comprehensive case management that was sometimes supplemented by intensive counseling. The extent of intervention by staff depended upon factors such as the family's own capacity to access the service, the complexity of intake procedures at the provider agency to which referral was being made, and the number of services requested.

The number of referrals made by the project is an illuminating measure of the unmet service needs of this population. A total of 328 referrals were made to other services and resources: 37% were to different types of respite services under other auspices such as in-home, day care, and institutional facilities; 23% to social service agencies for socialization programs, in-home services, intensive or prolonged counseling, housing, and financial entitlements; 12% to medical services; 8% to self-help groups; 7% to diagnostic centers; and 5% to legal services. Those statistics do not adequately portray the range and diversity of caregiver service needs, however. Within those categories were referrals for free diapers, medical care, cleaning services, legal services, financial entitlements, long-term care homemakers, medical equipment, case management, transportation, nursing homes, self-help support groups, advocacy groups, and senior citizen groups.

When referrals did not fully meet the family's needs, the project staff provided case management service, including advocacy, service monitoring, and reassessment.

> A caregiver was referred to the Area Agencies on Aging (AAA) Long-Term Care system for help with bathing her husband. Due to the complexity of the system and the caregiver's uncertainty about using help, the social worker checked weekly. Once the service began and the caregiver was satisfied, the worker reduced her involvement to monthly calls. Four months after the service began, the caregiver canceled the service because the agency had changed the time of day for the bath to the late afternoon. The worker intervened with the agency on behalf of the caregiver, and service was reinstated to the morning time that had proved satisfactory.

> Mr. and Mrs. G., both in their mid-eighties, lived in a rundown, dirty, three story house in an unsafe section of the city. Mrs. G., the caregiver, had emphysema and glaucoma. Her husband was incontinent and noncommunicative. A son who lived more than two hours away visited monthly at which time he did

grocery shopping, bathed his father, and periodically took his mother to doctors. Mrs. G. wanted help, but didn't want "a lot of people in her home at the same time." The FRCP social worker involved an AAA in-home social worker and together they planned to solve the family's multiple problems one by one. Chore service was obtained to clean the house so as to decrease the dust that aggravated Mrs. G.'s emphysema. Following the general clean up, living space in the house was rearranged so that Mr. and Mrs. G. could live solely on the first floor. Next, a homemaker was secured from the AAA twice weekly for two hours each time to bathe Mr. G., assist with laundry, and dust the first floor. The AAA arranged for medical transportation for biweekly medical visits for Mrs. G., while the FRCP social worker arranged respite to coincide with these appointments. Finally, Mrs. G. agreed to use the time the homemaker was in the home to visit a friend on the street occasionally.

Counseling

Counseling helped clients with their distressing feelings about the caregiving situations and with interpersonal or personal problems that may have been inhibiting their use of respite service. Three-fifths of the caregivers received such counseling, the form and content of which was, of course, as diverse as their characteristics and situations.

In most instances, counseling was short term with two-fifths of the recipients receiving counseling for less than two months, and slightly more than half for two to five months. Five percent of the families received the service for six or more months, and a small group received sustained counseling during the entire project year. The amount as well as the duration of the counseling also varied, ranging from less than an hour to nine hours during the project year. In some situations, the need for counseling exceeded the scope of the project. About 7% of the caregivers had long-term intensive counseling needs, were receptive to referrals for psychotherapy, and were referred to private practitioners, family service agencies, and PGC's Counseling for Caregivers program.

The content of the counseling also varied. A major problem for many caregivers was that they were unaware that their feelings and reactions were "normal." They needed reassurance from staff about their feelings being natural, acceptable, and experienced by others in similar situations. The understanding conveyed by a professional relieved them and encouraged more in-depth sharing of emotions that could be dealt with in the counseling process. Many caregivers were unable to use respite until they had been helped to express their anxieties, fears, and negative feelings about the patient.

As part of the counseling process, some questions were asked (these questions were not part of the research protocol used for both the experimental and control groups) that served to "normalize" issues about which some caregivers feel embarrassed. For example, prefacing certain questions with the statement "We find that caregivers often have problems with X, do you experience . . . ?," freed them to realize that they were not alone in having "secrets" such as alcohol use, sexual intimacy with the impaired person, or wishes for the latter's death.

Many caregivers who were initially reluctant to use respite were enabled to do so by the counseling process. Such reluctance is a pervasive theme in reports of respite demonstrations. For other clients, reluctance is better described as resistance that failed to yield to counseling despite their clear need. The discussion below focuses first on situations in which counseling resulted in use of respite. Nonusers of respite and the reasons for nonuse are then described.

Some participants required ongoing counseling support to use and continue to use respite. Some felt too depleted to undertake a new experience, one that sometimes generated fear and frustration. Making plans, leaving a loved one in the care of a stranger, or preparing the patient to attend day care posed both emotional issues and patient management problems.

> Mr. S. was reluctant to try respite because his wife became upset when left with strangers. At the social worker's suggestion, he agreed to bring an aide into the house on two separate occasions while he was at home, in order to familiarize Mrs. S. with a new person. On the third occasion he left the house for an

hour, on the fourth occasion for two hours, and on the fifth for four hours. The plan was successful because both Mr. and Mrs. S. were able to get used to the new situation slowly.

Mrs. N. desperately wanted respite but was fearful of leaving her mother because the latter was always agitated and hard to manage. With the social worker's encouragement, Mrs. N. began to keep a daily log noting the patient's quieter times. As expected, a pattern of "quiet times" emerged and in-home respite was successfully arranged to coincide with those times.

At times, caregivers needed counseling to validate their troubling experience before they felt "entitled" to respite services. When successful, this was a particularly gratifying aspect of the counseling process. Staff were able to encourage caregivers to try respite for a special one-time event: "Try it once and see how it works for you." The good experience often resulted in more use of respite service.

Ms. J. had been caring for her severely impaired mother for five years. She was emotionally and physically exhausted and had not seen her friends or participated in any social activities for over a year. Because she worked full-time and her mother received day care at PGC, Ms. J. felt she was not entitled to additional time away from her mother. The focus of counseling was to validate Ms. J.'s difficulty in working and caregiving concurrently, and to identify the "normal" need for leisure time. When a weekend business trip that could be combined with visiting a friend was offered to Ms. J., she agreed to try it. She arranged institutional respite at the PGC with subsidy support and returned from her weekend trip feeling better than she had in years. As a result, she planned monthly outings for which she herself paid.

While counseling helped those caregivers who felt too overwhelmed to partialize the problems and begin to explore solutions, most of them moved very slowly towards acceptance of respite. Often, problems such as financial hardship, patient management difficulties, and conflicted relationships with the patient and other family members were sorted out one by one before respite was used.

GOSHEN COLLEGE LIBRARY
GOSHEN, INDIANA

Perhaps most difficult were the situations in which the caregiver's own needs were tightly bound to the needs of the patient. Typically, such caregivers were older, isolated women who had been caring for their spouses for many years. The casework focus was to help them recognize their own needs and interests as legitimate and as separate from those of the patient, and to envision some life of their own. It was difficult for them to grasp the concept that the instrumental tasks of caregiving were not inextricably bound to the love and support they provided and that the former could be accomplished (even if not as well) by others. These problems were compounded when the caregivers had no outside interests or place to go, and required particularly creative case-work intervention.

> Elderly Mrs. K. had been caring for her severely demented husband for more than six years. The only other family member lived 1500 miles away. The caregiver never went out of the home and the social worker was able to identify only one interest: cooking. After much case work, the social worker struck a bargain with Mrs. K. She would allow Mrs. K to teach the social worker how to cook an ethnic dessert if, at the time for the lesson, an aide could be brought in to watch Mr. K. The successful outcome was that the social worker then was able to involve Mrs. K. in a cooking class in a local community center's senior citizen group.

Counseling was needed almost invariably when nursing home placement was being considered. In some cases, helping families to use respite later evolved into a process of helping them think things through in relation to institutionalization of the patient. Even when the caregiver could no longer manage at all and was under severe strain, the prospect of placement stimulated a complex of feelings such as guilt, conflict, anxiety, fear, and despair.

> Mrs. J. was devoted to her mother, for whom she had been caring for four years. The mother required constant attention because she was frequently agitated, sometimes incontinent,

and awake most nights. Even though she was exhausted and depressed, Mrs. J. was reluctant to use respite assistance, feeling that no one could care for her mother as well as she. When Mrs. J.'s daughter, who lived in another city, had a baby, the social worker encouraged her to visit her new granddaughter. With social worker support, Mrs. J. explored a nursing home respite stay for her mother. The visit with her daughter and new grand-daughter was successful: Mrs. J. returned refreshed. She also was pleased with how her mother's one-week stay in the nursing home had gone—her mother had been well-cared for and the nursing home staff had been pleasant and caring.

Two months later the situation had deteriorated. A visit to Mrs. J.'s home revealed that the mother was incontinent of both bowel and bladder. The caregiver was overwhelmed, exhausted, and depressed. She could not keep up with the house and her mother. In-home respite was immediately arranged and the social worker began to discuss with Mrs. J. the possibility of institutionalizing the mother. The social worker recognized Mrs. J.'s love and devotion to her mother, yet at the same time separated emotional caring from physical caring. The excellent physical care the mother received during the nursing home respite day was recalled. With sensitive counseling, Mrs. J. began to explore long-term placement, and the mother eventually was placed in a nursing home.

Crisis intervention was another form of counseling used. The project identified particularly vulnerable families that needed a sustained connection with the worker not only in relation to use of respite but because they were at risk of emergencies. The relationships with project social workers established a climate in which the families turned to them for help in times of crisis, whether or not they had received respite service.

The situation of Mrs. T., a mentally limited caregiver, erupted into a full-blown crisis. She had called the social worker to report that her husband was sleeping too much and she was frustrated and tired of him. The social worker visited immediately and found that Mr. T. required emergency medical treatment. Mrs. T. initially was adamant in refusing to allow him to be hospitalized. Due to the strong relationship with the social worker that had developed, she finally agreed to hospitalization.

Family group counseling was provided to about 10% of the families in order to help caregivers share information with their families and to try to enlist their help. When families were receptive, staff participated in family meetings to educate them about disease symptoms and progression, ways to manage problem behaviors, and the problems experienced by the caregivers in coping with the situation. The other family members were encouraged to share decisions about respite plans or long-term care plans and to participate in resolving crisis situations. In addition, the family meetings aimed to resolve intrafamilial relationship problems that had been exacerbated by the caregiving situation.

During the initial interview it became clear that Mrs. D. was denying her frustration with caring for her husband. Because Mr. D. had not been diagnosed by a physician, Mrs. D. was hampered in understanding, accepting, and planning for the problems she faced. In the past Mr. D. had been a strong leader of the family, and his wife was accustomed to following his directions. Now she was floundering. The D's daughter had withdrawn from her parents because of frustration with her mother's unwillingness to see the need for help. Mrs. D. refused our initial offer of respite, saying that she was managing well. The social worker recommended that a diagnostic work-up be done and suggested several possible medical centers. Mrs. D. was also given literature and an explanation of dementia and its course in order to help her to begin thinking about a long-range plan for her husband.

Several weeks later, FRCP received an emergency call from the daughter saying that Mrs. D. had packed a bag, left her husband, and was calling the daughter from a phone booth a mile from home. At the social worker's suggestion, the daughter went to her parents' home and met with Mrs. D. and a granddaughter to discuss the long-term consequences of Mr. D.'s mental impairment, the immediate and future difficulties of caring for him, and steps that could be taken to ease the burden for Mrs. D. Though Mrs. D. has no specific plans to use respite services, as a result of FRCP's intervention she made an appointment for a diagnostic work-up for her husband and her daughter persuaded her to go out for an evening concert—a treat Mrs. D. had not enjoyed in years.

In summary, *counseling was the linchpin service* that enabled some caregivers to use respite and helped them in many other ways as well. Counseling assisted participants:

- to resolve and accept negative feelings towards the impaired person;
- to recognize that they were "entitled" to leisure time and a life of their own;
- to sort out their own needs from those of the impaired person;
- to try something new (respite) and work out the problems involved in getting and using help;
- to partialize and solve problems that inhibited the use of services;
- to resolve crisis situations;
- to recognize when they could no longer provide care and needed help;
- to plan long-term care; and,
- to involve their other family members in the caregiving situations.

NONUSERS OF FRCP RESPITE

While the case excerpts above described situations in which counseling was successful in enabling caregivers to use respite services, a substantial number of caregivers who were offered the services did not use them. (Data on rates of use of various types of respite will be presented in Chapter 4.)

Principal Reasons for Nonuse

There were several main categories of reasons for nonuse of the project's respite service:

Caregivers already receiving respite from other sources (formal or informal). Those receiving informal services typically had family members who made routine visits or arranged for specific periods of time when the caregiver needed relief.

Those receiving formal services prior to the project typically had located—rather then been located by—such services. Having identified the need on their own and armed with information provided by friends, doctors, staff of diagnostic services or of the Alzheimer's Association, they had made their own plans for relief. A small number of caregivers had come to the attention of social service agencies (in particular, the aging network), primarily because of the caregiver's vulnerability (the caregiver's own advanced age or poor health, for example). In most of these cases, however, the focus of the services was not specifically on respite. Rather, long-term care plans were made because the needs of the impaired person exceeded the family's capacity to manage; respite for the caregivers was a by-product of the plan. More of the small group of families who obtained nonproject respite did so because of referrals made by staff. During the life of the project, however, two local Area Agencies on Aging (AAA) (Philadelphia County and Delaware County) began to implement programs of in-home, day-care, and institutional respite.

Among the factors that differentiated project respite users from users of respite from other formal sources was the availability of subsidized services in the types, amounts and frequencies wanted by the family. Families found different ways of combining sources of help. A few families used both respite services from the project and those from the existing social service network and private sources. Often, a social service agency had stringent limits on the amounts and types of respite services, so that families' needs could be met only partially by that single agency. Families who could pay part of the cost often used private pay sources and the subsidized project respite.

Caregivers who appeared to manage without undue stress and did not use respite services of any kind. Among their reasons for refusing service were:

1. They did not feel the need for respite services because their patients were in the early stages of the disease and did not require constant supervision. The caregivers were still able to leave them to

care for their own medical needs, attend events, go to work, do household tasks, and pursue their own interests.

2. They stated that their patient was still too much aware of what was happening to feel comfortable in subjecting them to a temporary caregiving situation. At the other extreme, some felt quite comfortable leaving bedbound patients without any supervision for a couple of hours at a time.

3. They were caring for moderately to severely disabled patients, expressed satisfaction in providing care, and felt no need for relief. Many such people were interested in learning about respite options in case they might want to avail themselves of services in the future. Some did call on the project eventually.

4. Some caregivers had used respite unsuccessfully prior to the project and refused to try again. They reported that the lack of success had been due to unreliable and poor quality respite or that the patient's behavior became worse during and after respite use.

Caregivers who refused the service despite their views that they were not managing well and could benefit from respite. This group is of particular concern because it included some of the most vulnerable caregivers—those in poor health, with severely limited finances, and with minimal family or friend support. There were two main reasons for this refusal: cultural attitudes they held about caregiving, and psychological barriers.

BARRIERS TO USE OF RESPITE SERVICES

Cultural Attitudes and Refusal of Respite

With respect to attitudes about caregiving, it is important to note that respite care is a new concept and service, a societal response to the radical demographic changes of the past few decades. The new response recognizes that eldercare is a social as well as family responsibility. Many caregivers, however, still hold attitudes about caregiving that were formed many decades ago. Thus, they frequently refuse respite services because they believe that it is their responsibility alone to provide the care, or that persons of their ethnic, racial or religious group "take care of their own."

> Ms. J., a widow in her early 70s, has been caring for her severely impaired mother for three years despite her own health problems. There was no family on whom she could rely for assistance. She was steadfast in her refusal of respite services. "My mother took care of her mother, and now it is my turn to care for her. She did it, so can I. [Her ethnic group] always take care of their own." A social worker's attempts to differentiate the two situations—that is, the mother had been younger and in better health when called upon for caregiving and the mother's siblings provided help—were to no avail.

This attitude about caregiving is compounded by the social norm of family responsibility. "Good families" are able to take care of each other, and for many people acceptance of outside help implies a loss of social status or power (Fulton & Katz, 1986). At times these attitudes are reinforced by extended family members who heighten the caregiver's resistance to respite services.

Psychological Needs and Refusal of Respite

Among the psychological barriers to use of FRCP's respite services was a pathological investment in not receiving assistance. Some caregivers were obviously enduring severe strains, but were so totally immersed in the caregiving role that they were unable to meet their own needs despite attempted intervention by family, friends, and project social workers. The litany of reasons expressed for not accepting respite included such statements as: "My mother took care of me," "My husband wouldn't want to be left with strangers," "Strangers aren't trustworthy," or "It's my job." Some such caregivers and their patients had had very poor relationships all their lives; the prospect of relief even for a short time stimulated severe guilt. Extensive counseling was unsuccessful in enabling them to use respite.

Among such caregivers were some who experienced difficulty in maintaining an identity separate from that of being the caregiver. Caregiving tasks can be totally consuming both in time and in emotional investment. As a result, some caregivers become so involved in meeting the disabled person's needs that their own needs for work, socialization, and leisure time become secondary or are ignored. They may reduce and even eliminate all other activities or fail to pursue interests outside of the caregiving role. Then, when respite is offered, they have nothing to do with their free time. Some consent to using respite to take care of household chores, but refuse service in order to have time to themselves or to have fun.

> Mrs. and Mrs. S. had been happily married and devoted to each other for 53 years. Mrs. S.'s dementia had recently progressed to the point where she required constant supervision and could not be managed outside of the home. Although Mr. S. expressed missing his weekly visit to the senior center, he refused respite service to attend. He explained to the social worker that attending the senior center had been something they had enjoyed as a couple. To attend and have fun without his wife would not be right. He was, however, willing to accept respite service when he visited the doctor.

The guilt that some caregivers experience despite the reality of their caregiving efforts also inhibits respite use. The caregiving situation in and of itself is fertile ground for evoking guilt. People struggle to be "good" caregivers and do the "right" thing for their relatives. Yet, the question as to what constitutes a "good" caregiver cannot be universally or easily answered. How much does one need to sacrifice and at what cost to one's self and one's family? Unrealistic expectations lead to feelings of failure. Those who believe that caregiving is their responsibility alone may feel conflicted and guilty about wanting respite. They may fear that something is wrong with them or with their ability to manage if they want a service that conflicts with their image of themselves as a good spouse or adult child. When there are competing time demands such as work or childcare, guilt may be stimulated or excerbated by the failure to do it all "well."

There are times in every caregiving situation when the caregiver experiences negative feelings about the impaired person and the situation. When such feelings (even wishing the person were dead) are unacceptable to the caregiver, again guilt can result. Some sense of guilt is almost universal, whether derived from caregivers' attitudes about their roles, how they evaluate their own competency, how others in the family regard them, or for other reasons. However, those caregivers in whom guilt is pervasive and severe often reject help because it intensifies their negative feelings or creates anxiety that something will happen to their loved one if left in the care of others.

> Mr. and Mrs. C. were eagerly anticipating Mr. C.'s retirement when it became necessary for Mrs. C.'s demented mother to come to live with them. The retirement plans were placed on hold. When approached by the respite social worker to try respite, Mrs. C. refused because she was afraid her mother would fall down the steps if left in another's care. With counseling, Mrs. C. confided to the social worker that she was horrified by her thoughts of wishing her mother would fall down the steps and die. Numerous counseling sessions focused on normalizing Mrs. C.'s negative thoughts and escape fantasies. However, Mrs. C. could not accept the negative thoughts about the mother she loved and refused respite assistance.

Some nonusers may be unable to adapt to the changes involved in using a new service. Change is difficult for people of every age, but it is even more difficult for caregivers whose behavioral patterns and attitudes about caring for family members may have prevailed for fifty years or more. Many caregivers have to cope with the multiple changes they and their relatives experience. Being thrust into another new situation—using an unfamiliar service—may be resisted. Leaving their helpless loved one in the care of strangers may produce severe anxiety.

The patients' behavioral problems also inhibit use of respite.

Mr. J., a 72-year-old caregiver, might have been receptive to in-home respite care for his wife. However, her daytime behavior of constant agitation and combativeness and nocturnal wandering exhausted him, depriving him of the energy to leave the house and created concern that a respite worker could not manage her. With the social worker's support, he tried numerous behavioral strategies to more effectively manage the behavioral symptoms and sought medication from a psychiatrist. Both interventions were partially successful in controlling her behavior, but she continued to be difficult to manage. In the end, Mr. J. decided to postpone respite until her behavior changed substantially.

Some families are overwhelmed by the complexity, difficulty, and time requirements of caregiving tasks. Moreover, the incidence of depression in caregivers (estimated to affect 50–75% of them) exacerbates feelings of being overwhelmed and depletes emotional resources. The initial time and emotional investment in arranging for respite services may require more energy than they can expend.

Mrs. D., who had been caring for her demented mother for three years, was overwhelmed and depressed. She reported to the social worker that she worried continuously, lacked the energy to adequately complete routine household tasks, and was going crazy staying in the house all the time. She had not been out in almost a year. When the social worker suggested that in-home respite would enable her to go out to meet with friends, she agreed to consider it, but became anxious about making all the arrangements. Over time, with the social worker's help, Mrs. D. was able to prepare for the outing. She decided when to go, called the respite agency to arrange the service, and prepared a list of information to review with the respite worker. On the day of the outing, the respite worker arrived 45 minutes late. Mrs. D. canceled the outing, saying she could not handle revising her plans. She refused all further suggestions of using respite.

Because caring for a mentally impaired older person entails watching that person deteriorate over time, caregivers often grieve and mourn the loss of their loved one or the prior relationship. Although each individual has a unique response to this situation, some may be too depressed to undertake anything new. For others, accepting respite may emphasize the change in the patient's status that they are trying to deny.

Ms. A., a 57-year-old widow, was devastated by her mother's diagnosis of Alzheimer's disease. Although she knew that something was wrong with her 83-year-old mother, she had delayed obtaining a diagnosis until her mother had wandered dangerously outside of their shared home while Ms. A. was grocery shopping. Ms. A. was fearful of leaving her mother alone and was unable to do her errands and visit her friends. Although initially receptive to the social worker's suggestion to explore day-care respite, she returned from the visit to the day-care center upset and adamantly opposed to using it. She perceived that the day care participants were very impaired and they scared her mother. Through discussion, the social worker learned that in reality Ms. A.'s mother had not expressed any negative feelings about the visit and the participants were by and large similar to Ms. A.'s mother. Despite counseling, Ms. A. remained unable to fully acknowledge that her mother had Alzheimer's disease, and refused day-care respite.

System Barriers to Respite Use

A major obstacle to use of respite are barriers presented by the formal system of health care services of which respite services are a part. The formal system is a discontinuous and fragmented system (Brody, Poulshock, & Masciocchi, 1978), with the various service components not being related to or coordinated with each other. Each service has its unique eligibility criteria, that is, age, income, medical status, residency, length-of-service criteria, costs, and access patterns. To secure most services, a family must first identify its specific needs and know about and seek out the appropriate service(s). There is no universal case management service that identifies needy individuals and assists their access to and utilization of services. As disabled persons move from one level of care to another, services are simply discontinued for one level and not automatically given at the next. It is a baffling system for professionals and families alike, requiring sophistication, motivation, and perseverance.

An additional obstacle encountered during this study was that the available respite services are perceived by some caregivers as nonacceptable. Complaints about in-home respite workers related to the latter's unreliability, lack of motivation, or lack of knowledge about caring for mentally impaired persons adequately. Some families found that being unable to rely on a respite worker arriving at the arranged time was more than they could tolerate. For caregivers living with impaired persons whose behavior was unpredictable, the level of uncertainly was increased.

Many barriers that the service system presents to the utilization of respite services (see Chapter 1) were not experienced by caregivers in this study because the service model was designed to minimize those barriers. Project staff encountered such barriers, however, when they tried to access nonproject respite services.

Financial Barriers to Respite Use

A common theme in this and other respite studies (e.g., Duke University Aging Center) is the reluctance of many families to use their financial resources for respite until "they really need it"—that is, until they are physically and emotionally depleted. In addition, they fear that if they exhaust their resources for community care, funds will not be available for nursing home care if that time should come. When services are offered without cost or for modest fees, some caregivers are reluctant to accept "charity" or do not wish to subject themselves to public disclosure of income and demeaning means testing.

Many fee-for-service respite options, (i.e., day care, institutionalization, and in-home services) did exist in Philadelphia at the time of the project. However, they were not affordable for those whose incomes were low, and fee-for-service respite severely strained the finances of people with moderate or middle incomes. The latter were excluded by existing publicly funded services that were generally targeted to the poor or

near-poor. These publicly funded services were extremely
scarce. The demands for service far exceeded the resources
available, so that people languished on waiting lists or received
only part of what they required.

Another financial barrier encountered by the project staff
was the sliding scale to determine family payment in existing
programs. Although families want to and do receive services on
a cost-sharing basis, many sliding scale formulae were the
same ones used to determine eligibility for child-care or couples programs and were too stringent. The issues and the commitment of resources for eldercare are quite different. For
example, older couples may be resistant to spending money for
respite because they want to conserve their resources in case
nursing home placement is needed later. Caregiving adult children may be supporting their own children's education or trying to save for their own impending retirement. An unresolved
dilemma is whether the older person's resources or the caregiver's resources should be taken into account in computing
contributions.

Most publicly funded programs use the care recipient's functional impairment level as a criterion for eligibility. This dis-
criminates against caregivers who are desperate for relief but
whose patients are in the mid stage of Alzheimer's disease and
do not meet the eligibility criteria.

In some publicly funded programs, the procedures to secure
respite are cumbersome and intrusive. In one Area Agency on
Aging for example, caregivers desiring subsidy for day care
were required to submit to two complete assessments at home
by two workers before even getting to the day-care center to
ascertain whether day care was appropriate. In another program, caregivers had to pay the respite provider before being
reimbursed, rendering this program unavailable to the poor. In
still another program the respite subsidy changed monthly,
thereby creating the need for devising respite arrangements
every month. Many caregivers refused to participate in such
programs and the resistance of some to using respite increased.
Others, particularly those who were more vulnerable, simply
could not handle the extra burden.

To summarize this discussion on barriers to respite use, many caregivers (to a greater or lesser degree) hold attitudes and/or experience psychological dilemmas inherent in caregiving that are antithetical to respite use. Barriers in the formal system of services compound the problem and contribute to caregivers' resistance to using respite. On balance, the vast majority of families struggle against enormous obstacles to care for their dependent elderly. Some families are readily able to resolve such issues and use respite service; others require counseling before using respite. A small number, however, appear unable to resolve their conflicts and thus do not use and benefit from respite services.

The Research Design for Evaluating Respite Care

3

A major reason for the formation of the Multiservice Respite Program for Family Caregivers was to provide an opportunity for evaluating the effects of respite intervention. Most of the details of the research and the intricacies of some of the findings are of primary interest to other researchers. The purpose of this chapter is to provide enough information on the evaluation to allow knowledgeable interpretation of the conclusions. The gerontological research literature will be the major source for the full presentation of these findings (Brody, Saperstein, & Lawton, 1989; Lawton, Brody, Saperstein, & Grimes, 1989: Lawton, Kleban, Moss, Rovine & Glicksman, 1989; Saperstein & Brody, in press).

THE STRUCTURE OF THE EVALUATION

The evaluation was planned as a randomized longitudinal experimental-control study. The essential requirement for such an evaluation is to constitute one group to experience the intervention and compare it with another group similar in every way but not given the intervention. Making the groups similar is best achieved by defining a total pool of eligible persons and randomly assigning half to the treatment group and half to the untreated control group. With a variation to be described later, this procedure was followed. The essential test of the effect of the intervention is performed by comparing the change observed in the treated group with that observed in the untreated group.

The Subjects: Families Caring for a Cognitively Impaired Older Relative

Although many types of disabilities require caregiving effort from families, the disability chosen for study in this project was that resulting from organic brain diseases typical of old age. These irreversible dementias included Alzheimer's disease, multi-infarct dementia and other forms of organic syndromes. Such diagnoses had been provided to the relative before the research began by a physician giving care to the older person.

The disabled older person had to be still living in the community (i.e., not in a nursing home, boarding home, mental hospital, congregate housing, or other institution).

The subject for the research was the primary caregiver of the older person. Such caregivers were self-identified and rarely was there a problem determining whether that relative was the primary caregiver. Any household living arrangement was acceptable, including those in which the caregiver and the impaired relative lived in different households.

Recruitment of Families

Respondents for the study came from five sources:

1. Self-help support groups of caregivers of Alzheimer's disease patients, sponsored by the Alzheimer's Association;
2. Volunteers who were made aware of the study through public service announcements by the media;

3. Referrals by service agencies (program descriptions were mailed several times to several hundred health and social service provider agencies);
4. Referrals by participants in the study; and
5. Referrals by professionals (e.g., doctors, social workers, nurses).

The most productive single source of caregivers was the network of Alzheimer's self-help groups. A total of 632 families were recruited and successfully completed the study, 295 of them from the support groups. The sample was thus a volunteer sample, rather than a representative sample. However, among the support groups 87% of the eligible families contacted agreed to participate.

Constituting the Experimental and Control Groups

Entire support groups were assigned randomly to the experimental or control programs. It was decided as a matter of ethics and public-relations to maintain the integrity of each support group, placing participants from any one group as whole units into either the experimental or control program. Because members of such support groups rely extensively on each other for emotional support, it was considered unwise to place members of the same support group into two different research programs (i.e., experimental and control groups). Volunteers or referrals from service agencies or others not associated with the study were randomly assigned as individuals to experimental and control programs.

The usual practice in randomized experiments is to inform potential respondents at the time they are recruited of the intent to assign volunteers randomly to experimental and control programs. We did not do so because the appeal made to potential participants was that they act as research volunteers in a study of caregiving, rather than to be potential recipients of respite service. An advertisement for people to test respite services would systematically bias the sample for a particular type of individual or situation. Thus, all participants expected initially to be interviewed only as research subjects.

All potential participants were assigned to experimental or control programs before they were contacted by the research teams, as a way of avoiding treatment bias affecting the baseline assessments. Persons assigned to the experimental program were not made aware of the availability of the project services until the baseline interview was completed. The experimental condition thus consisted only of the *offer* of the intervention, rather than necessarily receiving the treatment.

Timing of the Study

The study and the intervention lasted 12 months, with each participant expected to complete a pretest (baseline) interview and a posttest (Time 2) interview at the end of the one year study period.

The period of experimental study began upon completion of the pretest (baseline) interview and ended with termination procedures late in the twelfth month. The experimental program began immediately following the pretest and concluded 365 days later.

Face-to-Face Interviews:
The Baseline and Time 2 Evaluations

A face-to-face interview was the primary vehicle for gaining both the "pre" (baseline) and "post" (Time 2) data. Interviews were conducted in each caregiver's home (or occasionally elsewhere if requested by the caregiver) at a time when the respondent would be most free of distractions. Interviews were administered during one visit unless precluded by extreme circumstances, such as illness of an informant.

The baseline interview with the caregiver inquired about a variety of characteristics of the older person, the caregiver, and the context in which caregiving occurred:

- Background characteristics.
- The disabled older person's symptoms and behaviors.
- The types and amounts of assistance given by the caregiver.

- The types and amounts of assistance received from formal or paid sources.
- Assistance provided by other family members.
- Attitudes of the caregiver toward the caregiving task, including subjectively perceived burden, impact on social life, caregiving mastery, caregiving satisfactions, and caregiving ideology.
- Measures of the caregiver's health and mental health.

The interview typically lasted about 90 minutes.

The Time 2 follow-up interviews generally repeated baseline measures that might change, and added a number of sections on attitudes toward and evaluations of the services received over the 12 months (either experimental or spontaneously initiated nonexperimental services).

Because changes in the status of the impaired person occurred over the course of the year, the content of the Time 2 interview with the caregiver would differ depending on which of the following characterized the status of the impaired person after 12 months:

- Alive and residing in the community.
- Alive and residing in a nursing home.
- Deceased, having died while residing in the community.
- Deceased, having died while residing in a nursing home.

Thus, only caregivers whose patients were in the first of these four groups had a chance to be exposed to a full year of experimental respite services.

CHARACTERISTICS OF THE FAMILIES

Background Characteristics

In general, the random division of the subjects into experimental and control groups constituted two groups that were very similar. Their background characteristics are shown in Table 3.1. Not surprisingly, the impaired older person was more

Table 3.1. Characteristics of the Sample of Impaired Persons and Caregivers

The impaired person	Control group (percentage)	Experimental group (percentage)
Gender	63.4	55.9
Age (mean)	76.4	76.1
Marital status (% presently married)	45.7	56.2
Lives with primary caregiver	84.5	87.7
Education (% 13 or more years)	18.4	20.8
Mean cognitive symptom severity[a] (range 6–30)	13.7	12.7
Mean noncognitive severity[a] (range 17–65)	46.5	45.6
Primary caregiver		
Gender (% female)	77.9	80.8
Age (mean)	59.4	60.4
Marital status (%)		
Never married	7.9	7.3
Presently married	69.1	74.1
Widowed	7.6	8.8
Divorced or separated	15.5	9.7
Relationship to impaired person (%)		
Spouse	40.4	49.8
Child	41.3	35.9
Child-in-law	4.7	4.1
Sibling	4.7	3.8
Friend	2.2	1.6
Other	6.6	4.8
Racial background (% nonwhite)	22.1	28.7
Caregiver works (%)	35.2	33.1
Annual income (median)	14,600	14,500
Years of school (mean)	12.1	12.0

[a]High score denotes few symptoms

likely to be female, although this characteristic was very much a function of the relationship of the caregiving person: 85% of those being cared for by a child were female, while only 29% of those being cared for by a spouse were female. Caregiving by other than a spouse comes about only after the death of the spouse, resulting in the older-age pattern of an adult daughter caring for a widowed mother. About 85% of the caregiving was done by a spouse or other relative caregiver who shared a household with the impaired person.

Almost 80% of all caregivers were women. Eighty percent of spouse caregivers were over 65 but only 7% of adult-child caregivers were that old. Just under three-quarters (72%) were married. Forty-five percent were spouses, while 39% were adult children, and 16% were other relatives, with a few friends. The racial composition of the Philadelphia area was mirrored in the proportion of minorities (25% were black). About one-third of the caregivers were currently employed.

It was possible to compare these background characteristics with those of two larger and more broadly representative samples of caregiving families that have been reported in the literature, the National Long Term Care Survey (Stone, Cafferata, & Sangl, 1987) and the National Channeling Demonstration Study (Kemper, Brown, Carcagno, et al., 1986). For the most part, the respite sample was very similar to the others, although the Channeling study included a major group excluded by our sample—impaired older people who had no caregiver (33% of the Channeling sample). The major deviations of our sample from the national samples reflected the fact that our method of recruitment, conducted in a single major metropolitan area, resulted in people with a somewhat higher level of education and income than did the more representative samples. The median income of the caregiver in the respite sample was $14,500, that of the Channeling caregivers was $13,140; in education, 33% of the respite sample's caregivers had education beyond high school, as compared with 28% in the Channeling sample.

In summary, it must be emphasized that this was a volunteer sample and one which was very limited geographically. Therefore it would not be appropriate to claim that these respite findings can represent caregivers in general. In particular, the respite groups' higher-than-average socioeconomic status should be considered in relation to any generalization made from the present data. Deviations were minor in most other characteristics. Totally missing in our group of older Alzheimer victims, however, are the most deprived of the disabled elders, those with no identified caregiver.

THE THEORY OF CAREGIVING STRESS

Although the primary purpose of the research was to evaluate the effect of respite care, the research was guided by a theory of caregiving stress based on much of the previous work in this area, with elaborations that explored further the nature of the total set of gains and losses for the caregiver entailed in the process.

Lazarus and Folkman (1984) articulated a general theory of stress that guided our thinking in examining caregiving. Essential to this theory is the cognitive process by which a person assesses a situation in terms of its potential stressfulness ("primary appraisal"). One's coping efforts are shaped by the continuing appraisal of their adequacy and altered in response to the person's judgment about how well the coping is working ("secondary appraisal").

A perennial problem in stress research has been the distinction between objective and subjective stressor. Some feel that the distinction is specious, others (for example, Lazarus & Folkman, 1984) assert that in order for a situation to be a stressor, it must be appraised as stressful. This research pursued the idea that it was worthwhile to develop a measure of potential, or objective, stress, against which the appraised stress could be compared.

This conception thus began with the attempt to estimate objective stress in terms of the caregiving demand on the caregiver. Caregiving demand, in turn, was measured in terms of the *symptoms displayed by the impaired person*, that is, a rough indicator of the amount of attention and effort required of the caregiver. Beginning with the Problem Checklist of Zarit, Reever, and Bach-Peterson (1980), a list of possible symptoms of impaired people was developed. They included instances of cognitive failure such as disorientation and memory loss, socially deviant symptoms, and others. A factor analysis of items in the index yielded separate cognitive, social, and behavioral factors but the measure was used as a total symptoms score for the analyses (impaired-person symptoms).

We also felt that a different approach to defining objective stress was necessary to account for the fact that there would be substantial variation among caregivers in the extent of their responses to the same symptom pattern in the impaired person. For example, some would extend themselves greatly, others would be more sparing in their effort. Some would seek help from others, other caregivers would not seek help. Therefore we inquired extensively about the actual *amount of help provided by the caregiver*. Specifically, we inquired about the number of occasions per week and number of weeks in the year that help was given on 10 tasks of daily living. It was possible to sum such caregiving (using standard scores to take account of differences in the scales for each task) to arrive at an overall index of amount of care given. Amount of care provided may be called a "transactional" indicator of objective stress. That is, the amount of help given is a function of both the impaired person's disability (frequency of symptoms) and the caregiver's response, which would differ by reasons of capability to help and motivation to help.

Two other forms of help for the impaired person were seen as of potential importance in understanding the outcome of the caregiving process: The amount of *informal assistance* provided by other family, friends, or neighbors; and amount of *formal assistance* provided by agencies or paid help. For the varieties of personal assistance inquired about, the number of tasks for which help was provided by another informal helper was used as the measure of informal assistance (ranging from 0 to 9).

Amount of formal assistance was measured for six types of community-based services (homemaker, home-delivered meals, home health aide, home nurse, home professional rehabilitation, and transportation) plus the three forms of respite care (day care, in-home respite, and nursing-home respite). Units of service were defined for each service type; by asking about frequency of service units and the months during which the service was delivered it was possible to estimate the number of units of each formal service received during the year preceding the interview.

The amounts of objective stress (symptoms), care-giving effort by the caregiver, informal help received, and formal service received were, along with background characteristics (age and sex of the caregiver and impaired person, socioeconomic status, race, relationship to impaired person, living arrangement, and health of caregiver) hypothesized to affect the appraised stress experienced by the caregiver.

Although much has been learned about caregiving stress by using an indicator of overall stress or burden (e.g., the Burden Interview of Zarit et al., 1980), our theoretical orientation led us to differentiate among several subtypes of appraisal:

Subjective caregiving burden was an overall assessment, used in other research as well as in ours, evidenced by expressions of generalized worry, concern, and negative feelings about caregiving.

Caregiving satisfaction was a form of caregiving appraisal that we felt had been relatively neglected. A measure of this positive appraisal of the process of caregiving was thus developed for this research.

Caregiving mastery was an appraisal of the extent to which the caregiver and her caregiving efforts were judged to be competent and positive (related to secondary appraisal).

Caregiving impact on lifestyle was the extent to which the caregiver appraised her caregiving to have limited her freedom to engage in social and other types of activity.

Traditional caregiving ideology represents a person's appraisal of caregiving as an activity that fulfills important social and personal goals irrespective of how much it is liked or disliked.

We constructed our own measures of caregiving appraisal through factor-analytic techniques. Our hypotheses were that stronger stressors (more symptoms and more caregiving behavior) would increase negative appraisal and decrease positive appraisal, while assistance from others or from formal agencies would counteract these effects.

The ultimate outcomes selected for study were two aspects of mental health. *Depression* is the most frequently mentioned mental-health cost of caregiving; the Center for Epidemiological Studies Depression Scale (CESD, Radloff, 1977) was the measure used. In keeping with a great deal of research of the past two decades, it seemed important to represent positive mental health as well as depression. We therefore used the five-item *Positive Affect Scale* from the Bradburn (1969) Affect Balance Scale (ABS) as an indicator of feelings that are notable because they are better than average ("things going my way," "on top of the world," etc.).

George and Gwyther (1984) have argued that only mental health indicators such as the CESD and ABS should be used to assess programs like respite. The logic is that a measure that assesses anxiety or depression *about caregiving* explicitly is likely to mix up the stressor with the outcome—certainly an accurate criticism. Our approach differed in seeing the pathway that begins with caregiver and impaired person, and that ends with the mental health of the caregiver, as a channel of successive influences of one factor on another. That is, caregiving appraisal is itself an outcome of attributes of the caregiver, the impaired person, and the forms of assistance given and received. In turn, however, caregiving appraisal itself influences mental health. Most important, we suggest that depression and positive affect are also the result of some influences other than caregiving appraisal, such as the demographic characteristics and the health of the caregiver and the objective

stressors. In short we envisioned a causal model of the type
portrayed in Figure 3.1, in which an element to the left influences one or more of the elements to its right.

We added a feature to our model that built on previous
research that has shown negative and positive affective states
to have different antecedents (Bradburn, 1969; Lawton, 1983).
Specifically, we hypothesized that caregiving satisfaction
would elevate positive affect but have a less strong effect on
depression. Conversely, subjective caregiving burden should
increase depression but have a lesser effect on caregiving satisfaction. Further, we differentiated among the facets of caregiving appraisal in hypothesizing their antecedents. Specifically,
the amount of caregiving effort by the caregiver was hypothesized to increase subjective caregiving burden but, at the same
time, also to increase caregiving mastery and caregiving satis-

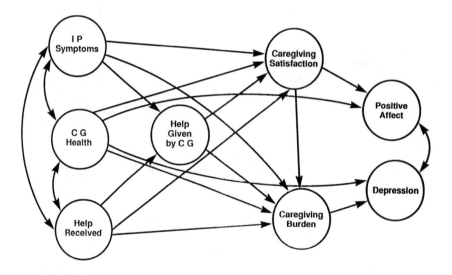

FIGURE 3.1 The dynamics of caregiving stress are hypothesized to
consist of influences from factors on the left operating directly or
through intermediate factors to result in outcomes to the right of the
influencing factor (influences indicated by arrows).

faction. This expectation was based on the idea that caregiving constitutes a challenge that may have diverse effects depending on the characteristics of the person. The demand to perform such tasks may well fortify the self (raise caregiving mastery) or provide self-enhancing feelings that one is doing right (caregiving satisfaction) even while the drudgery and unrelenting demands sustain a sense of worry (subjective burden).

THE ONE YEAR FOLLOW-UP STUDY

Regrettably, the meanings of most of the components of the caregiving stress model change depending on the course of the treatment year. There was considerable attrition during the research, with about 14% of the impaired people dying while living in the community before the end of the year, and 23% going to a nursing home. The major intermediate elements—caregiving time, formal and informal assistance, and caregiving appraisal—simply cannot be estimated and compared in a valid manner except among families whose older member was still alive and living in the community.

Thus the follow-up interviews, while all done about 12 months following baseline, were used for different research questions depending on the outcome group and the area of the inquiry. Chapter 4 will describe the research findings regarding the questions of who are the caregivers, what kinds of caregiving activities and services they experienced, and what types of respite services they used during the year. Chapter 5 will describe research findings on the effect of respite services, the effect of receiving respite services on caregiving activity and the use of formal services, and the test of the caregiving stress model.

Needs of Caregivers, Their Use of Services, and Their Caregiving Behavior

4

The caregiving families who volunteered for the respite research were not newcomers to the world of supportive services. Thus their uses of both respite and other services must be understood within the larger context of the needs of caregivers and their previous experiences with the service sector. This chapter, therefore, will begin with a discussion of some of the more prominent needs of caregivers. Data will then be presented on the original amount of use of services before the study began, followed by similar data on use of services over the 12 research months, including respite services. Barriers to the use of respite will then be discussed.

NEEDS OF CAREGIVERS

Caregiver needs may be viewed as falling into three categories: needs for expertise and support in caregiving, actual assistance in the process of caregiving, and the personal needs that happen to be served by performing care. The first category is most obvious—the needs are those associated with making their caregiving easier. Most caregivers begin with relatively little earlier experience caring for older people and, therefore need relevant knowledge about how to give care. An important feature of caregiver support groups involves sharing expertise about techniques that have worked. Group members also need help in understanding the condition of the impaired relative. The most popular visitor to the support group is a physician. Questions about the nature of chronic illnesses, the actions of pharmacologic agents, and the prospects for cure or ameliorative treatment are eagerly posed.

A second area of need is for actual assistance in the process of care. Although the general rule is that the spouse or one child, when available, or some other person, is the primary caregiver, there are few such primary caregivers who do not have some other forms of family assistance available. The other major form of help is the type given through formal service agencies, either nonprofit or proprietary, or through individual paid help. Our research group's uses of such services will be discussed in detail.

Personal needs of the caregiver, the third facet of need, are more diverse and harder to measure. Thus our data on personal needs are largely qualitative, some being generated by the anthropological interviews of our colleague Robert Rubinstein. The important feature of personal needs in relation to caregiving is that caregiving does something *for* the caregiver. As discussed earlier in relation to caregiving satisfactions, providing such care is by no means always an unmitigated burden.

One theme observed by many is the caregiver's perception of the justice of her giving care at this time. A typical expression is "My mother cared for me when I needed her; now it's my turn to care for her." This theme might be called the life-stage *caregiving equity* theme.

Another is also built on the idea that sharing the burden of caregiving is a felt duty that one wishes to pass along to one's children—the *caregiving modeling* theme. This view sometimes represents the caregiver's pride in continuing a family tradition of concern for elders. At the same time such a stance may be understood in exchange-theory terms—the sometimes not totally conscious thought that children may be more likely to provide care when needed by their parent when the parent has in turn set the example by caring for the grandparent.

Yet another personal need construes caregiving as an absolute religious or *moral imperative*. Authority is sought in the Bible, in lifelong religious teaching, or in a humanistic ethical code.

A different family of personal needs is based more clearly in a balance of gains and losses for the caregiver. One of the most frequent themes is caregiving as an *ego challenge*: Performance of the required tasks constitutes a test of personal competence. Related to the challenge theme is the view of caregiving as an important stage of adult development for some people. Caregiving is seen by some people as one of the developmental tasks whose successful performance leads the person into a more mature stage of life. It is not, of course, developmental in the sense of being either universal or inevitable. Nor is it developmental in that it occurs in the same stage of life for all caregivers. To the contrary, caregivers' stages of life vary widely, ranging from young adulthood to old age. But for those who perform the task, caregiving is frequently construed as a stage in their own lives.

Some caregivers' needs may be to maintain *continuity* for themselves within their social context. Familial roles such as "mother's favorite," "the burden bearer," "the responsible one," "the entertainer" become learned; performance of these roles may be an important source of security. Thus for some, the role of caregiver may represent the continuation of a lifelong role, where the person gains from the continuity but also experiences pressure to maintain that role through the expectations of others who expect that role's performance. Thus, continuity may have elements of both choice and compulsion.

Some may be quite overt in their experiencing of lifelong and/or current resentment of parental demands, yet continue the caregiving pattern in either resignation or triumph: "I'll endure it in the knowledge that I'll be free some day" or "I'll show her that I'm not easily cowed."

All such themes may serve to provide meaning to the caregiver's life and ultimately to strengthen the sense of competence of the stressed person. The themes are relevant to understanding people's specific behaviors in relation to the way they care for their impaired relative and the kinds of assistance they seek and use.

The foregoing is not to suggest that every caregiver's life is composed of positive ego-maintaining content. Rather, this recounting of needs that are positively served by caregiving is meant to moderate the view much more prevalent in our society that caregiving is an unmitigated burden. Our research data are consistent with those of others who have assessed the burdensome side of caregiving. The median score of our sample on a depression measure (Center for Epidemological Studies Depression scale, CESD, Radloff, 1977) was exactly at the level marking the beginning of the clinical depression range established for the population at large. In other words, half of our caregivers would be characterized as "depressed" by comparison with a representative sample of all adults. Few caregivers report a total absence of burden, but just as few appear to experience the demands of caregiving as a stressor strong enough to precipitate a major psychiatric illness. It is necessary, therefore, to view caregiving as a mixture of uplifts and hassles (Lazarus & Folkman, 1984), satisfactions and burdens. The actual behavior of people as they use or avoid using services may be understood better in light of what we might call the "mixed bag" experience of caregiving.

USE OF SERVICES AT BASELINE

It is important to know the extent of caregiving operations at baseline, how the level of such behaviors changed over the year of service, and how such changes may have varied with the status changes of the impaired person over that year. This section will present detailed data on the receipt of formal services, the amounts of assistance provided by the primary caregiver, and the prevalence of assistance from informal caregivers other than the primary caregiver. Finally, the actual amounts of respite care provided will be considered.

Formal Supportive Services

Table 4-1 shows the percentages of subjects who received each of six community-based supportive services at baseline, either from social agencies, proprietary agencies, or from private sources. "Sitter" services were not included in the baseline inquiry; shopping assistance was included but occurred so rarely that it is not presented here. These percentages denote families who used a service one or more times in the year before baseline.

About one-third of all families used the home-health aide or other paid personal-care assistance, in-home nursing or other medical treatments, and transportation services. Less frequent were homemaker, and therapeutic services (occupational therapy, physical therapy, speech therapy, and others), while home-delivered meals were very infrequent.

Informal Assistance

Shown in Table 4.2 are the percentages for the experimental and control groups who reported having been helped by another family member or other informal source in performing some of the basic assistance tasks. Transportation was the only service for which even half received such help. For the

Table 4.1. Percentage Using Community Services Before Treatment

Service	E	C
Homemaker	15.6	27.8
Home-delivered meals	5.7	5.4
Home health aide	39.4	36.6
Visiting nurse	34.3	30.9
OT, PT, speech therapy	14.9	15.1
Transportation	30.8	36.9

Table 4.2. Percentage of Caregivers Receiving Assistance from Other Informal Sources

Service	E	C
Transportation	52	56
Medication	19	28
Financial	22	22
Feeding	30	33
Dressing	19	23
Grooming	22	28
Toileting	17	20
Ambulation	14	21
Bathing	18	21

other critical activities of daily living, between 14% and 33% received help one or more times during the previous year. Such data, when compared to similar rates representing the caregiving performed by the primary caregiver, confirm the central position held by that primary caregiver. Help from secondary caregivers represents a relatively small amount of all care.

Respite Services

In assessing the overall volume of respite services received, it is important to note that two types of assistance were provided by secondary caregivers: (1) respite care for the primary caregiver, and (2) personal and instrumental care provided to the impaired person. For each secondary caregiver we systematically inquired about and obtained the number of hours of care in both categories, thus obtaining overall estimates of hours per year of respite care and personal and instrumental care received from secondary caregivers.

Explicit reports were also obtained about the number of hours per year of paid respite care, and the number of occasions and hours of day care, the use of nursing homes, acute hospitals, and boarding homes, and the number of days of respite care in institutes.

Table 4.3 shows the percentages of controls and experimentals who reported having received each of the two types of informal respite and the three major modes of formal respite service during the twelve-month period before the study began. Table 4.3 also shows the actual numbers who used each service, the median number of hours used by those who used the service, and the mean number of hours reported, averaged over both those who used and those who did not use the service. These data show, first, that the small amounts of specific ADL assistance given by secondary caregivers, when cumulated, did provide some relief for a majority of primary caregivers. The annual total, over 300 hours per year, includes help given by other household members, which consistently increases the overall average. Second, even greater percentages (64% of the experimental group and 75% of the control group) had specific respite occasions provided by secondary caregivers.

Table 4.3 also shows the baseline levels of formal respite services—in-home respite, day care, and nursing-home respite. Such services were, of course, far less prevalent than informal respite, but it is of great interest to see that well over one-third had already availed themselves of respite services. The combination of formal and informal community-based assistance, including respite, was clearly not at a negligible level for these caregivers.

THE TASKS PERFORMED BY
THE PRIMARY CAREGIVERS

Most caregiving research has used some measure of the amount of caregiving assistance provided by the caregiver. Such measures are often based on a count of the number of activities requiring help or on some average or aggregate estimate of number of hours per week. The present research attempted to measure in much greater detail than usual the actual amounts of assistance given. The task seemed hopeless, however, if the request was made to estimate actual time spent

Table 4.3. Respite Use, Year Before Baseline[a]

Service	Controls				Experimentals			
	Percentage using	N	Median	X̄ (all subjects)	Percentage using	N	Median	X̄ (all subjects)
Paid respite hours	31.6	100	168	275.6	27.9	88	164.5	148.8
ADL hours (informal)	70.3	223	170	335.4	55.9	176	136	308.4
Respite hours (informal)	75.4	237	264	543.7	64.4	203	168	345.7
Day care hours	19.9	63	409	111.1	19.4	61	196	85.8
Nursing home respite days	1.8	6	8	.17	0.9	2	b	b
Total number of services		317				315		

[a]Percentage and number of subjects who used each type of respite, median amount of use among all who used, and mean amount of use among all subjects (users and nonusers).
[b]Numbers too small for reliable estimate.

in each of a list of caregiving activities. People conceive of such tasks much more easily in terms of their frequency. Although the length of time for each occasion varies widely across occasions and by caregiver or disabled person, an instance of help with bath, eating, or transportation is likely to average out into some "usual" length of time for each unit as the instances are aggregated. This research inquired about whether assistance had ever been given during the past year for 10 different activities. If help had been given, people were then asked to say over how many of the 12 months such help had been given and the number of times per day, week, or month that help had been given. Table 4.4 shows these data for the control and experimental groups. (Data for such tasks as cooking, housekeeping, and laundry were obtained but are not presented because people found it difficult to estimate how much extra time performing such activities required in order to provide care to the impaired person.) The data show that somewhat over half required help with toileting and somewhat fewer than half required help in getting around the house. Help with all other activities was much more frequent and had been required the majority of the year. The mean number of occasions per month are shown; a few activities, such as providing help with toileting and getting around the house, were performed by some people with extraordinarily high frequencies and others with very low frequencies, so the averages tend to be inflated by the high-frequency users.

It is clear that the group of volunteer caregivers was performing tasks requiring an immense amount of time and effort. Many caregivers had assistance from others and also found help from formal agencies, but the bulk of the caregiving was provided by their own efforts.

THE RESEARCH YEAR: SERVICES RECEIVED

The way experimental services were provided has been described in Chapter 2. The control subjects, as well as experimental subjects, were contacted regularly in order to gather

Table 4.4. Amounts and Frequencies of Help Given by Caregiver—Baseline ($N = 632$)

Help given	Control group			Experimental group		
	Percentage giving help	Mean		Percentage giving help	Mean	
		Mo. helped	X/mo.		Mo. helped	X/mo.
Transportation	84.5	10.36	12.79	87.0	9.91	11.65
Take medicine	89.3	10.35	71.51	85.1	10.93	74.60
Finances	88.0	11.55	6.68	86.7	11.50	5.13
Eat	74.1	10.27	69.39	74.0	9.99	79.00
Dressing	83.9	10.32	51.17	82.5	10.46	52.60
Grooming	79.5	10.58	35.10	77.8	10.58	30.92
Toileting	56.2	10.00	115.98	62.9	9.87	105.90
Get around home	42.9	9.70	143.68	43.8	9.88	116.53
Bath	79.2	10.25	21.60	78.4	10.41	25.39
Shopping	79.6	10.28	7.55	76.3	10.21	61.38

data on their status, that is, whether the disabled person had moved, entered an institution, or died. Questions about service needs were answered for control families by referring them to the resource guide or the local information and referral agency. Thus, any services used by the control families during the research year were procured on their own, while experimental subjects could have had repeated help and encouragement by the respite project's professional staff.

This section of the report will examine the separate histories of service use for experimental and control families in terms of formal agencies and explicit respite services. It will also look again at the caregiving activities of the primary caregiver and the assistance obtained from informal secondary caregivers during the research year.

First, however, it is necessary to describe the outcomes for the 632 subjects over the course of the 12 research months. The number available for follow-up study was reduced to 558 because of moves, refusals, deaths of caregivers, and changes of caregivers. Sixty-three percent of the patients were still living in the community a year after baseline, 14% had died while living in the community, and 23% had entered a nursing home, of whom 20% had died there (overall death rate of 19%). Although all caregivers were interviewed a year after baseline, the amount of service use during the year is meaningful primarily for those families whose older person lived the entire year in the community. Except for the experimental respite use, other formal and informal service use will be described for only the community-alive group.

Table 4.5 shows the percentages of the community-alive group who used each type of service during the service year. In general, the control group was fairly stable in its use of formal service, decreasing about 7% in its use of in-home therapeutic visits and increasing slightly in homemaker and transportation use. The experimental group increased its use of formal services more widely—16% more used homemaker services, 9% more home health, 17% more transportation. The amounts of services used were also tracked; they are shown in Table 5.5 and discussed in Chapter 5. Social support services such as

Table 4.5. Percentages Using Formal Services at Baseline and Time 2 (Community-Alive Only)

Service	Control		Experimental	
	BL	T2	BL	T2
Homemaker	22	30	19	35
Home meals	4	5	6	10
Home health aide	30	35	35	44
Home nurse	28	28	28	29
Home therapy	17	10	11	12
Transportation	33	43	25	42

$N = 174$ for control group; 177 for experimental group.

home health/personal care and transportation were very frequent for those who used them at all, while technical services such as in-home therapy and home nursing were least frequently used.

Respite Services During the Research Year

Families in both the experimental and control groups were free to locate and obtain any kind of service on their own, even respite services. This section will describe the total amounts of respite used by the 350 community-alive families. Table 4.6 shows baseline and Time 2 respite use for the 173 controls and the 177 experimental living in the community 12 months later. The controls showed an increase in all forms of respite. The experimental subjects showed not only the expected increases in amounts of formal respite but also in amount of informal respite.

Respite Care: The Experimental Program

Turning to experimentally provided respite care, the amounts of use made by all experimental subjects will be considered first (that is, not just the community-alive group). Despite the fact that every family was offered respite and encouraged

Table 4.6. Amounts of Respite Use, Baseline and Time 2: Community Alive

	Controls			Experimentals		
Baseline	N	Median	X̄ (all Subjects)	N	Median	X̄ (all subjects)
Paid respite hours	49	165.5	279.3	42	288	135.2
ADL hours (informal)	124	152	349.3	99	135	278.5
Respite hours (informal)	135	265	599.7	111	142	355.0
Day care hours	31	432	104.5	31	96	63.2
Nursing home respite days	1	—	—	0	—	—
Time 2						
Paid respite hours	59	242	411.5	103	190	383.9
ADL hours (informal)	105	156	334.2	110	222	293.7
Respite hours (informal)	135	220	675.5	114	246	466.6
Day care hours	43	490	151.6	67	540	223.8
Nursing home respite days	5	(20)	(.52)	17	12	1.11

$N = 173$ for Control group, $N = 177$ for Experimental group.

87

periodically to consider whether it was needed, only about half (51.6%) ever availed themselves of the offer.

Patterns of use varied widely. To gain an idea of both amount of use and how the use was spread over time, Table 4.7 displays the types, amounts, and duration of various respite services given by the experimental respite program. It should be noted that the total N of 322 includes a few cases that were dropped during the service year for a variety of reasons such as refusals to participate further and missing research data.

The overwhelming majority of families who used respite— 67% of them—chose only in-home respite, while 14% chose institutional respite only, 4% chose day care only, and 15% used a combination of those services.

It is important to note that agency subsidies for in-home and institutional respite were practically nonexistent in the Philadelphia area when the experimental respite program began. Initially, subsidized day care respite was also generally unavailable. However, during the research year four new day care centers were opened and subsidies for day care respite were offered through the local Area Agency on Aging. Because our project staff referred caregivers for those subsidies, many fewer caregivers relied on the experimental program for day care subsidies than might otherwise have been the case.

In-Home Respite

In-home respite proved to be the form of respite most acceptable to the families. The main type of in-home help used was homemaker service. Such workers are generally employed by agencies and have limited or no training in health related matters. These homemakers functioned as companions who also could assist with tasks such as cooking and household maintenance. Home health care aides certified by Medicare home health care agencies were used to a lesser extent. They too performed tasks such as supervision, companionship, and IADL assistance, but also helped with ADL functions such as dressing, grooming and bathing the patient.

Table 4.7. Use of Respite Care Services by Experimental Subjects (Total N = 322): Duration of Use and Hours/Days Used

Length of time service used:	Those using In-home respite (N = 136)		Those using day care (N = 12)		Those using nursing home respite (N = 44)	
	N	Percentage	N	Percentage	N	Percentage
10 or more months	14	10.3	2	16.7	—	—
7 to 9 months	15	11.0	0	—	—	—
3 to 6 months	50	36.8	4	33.3	3	6.8
less than 3 months	57	42.0	6	50.0	41	93.2
Total persons using:						
100 or more hours	49	36.0				
75 to 99 hours	13	9.6				
50 to 74 hours	20	14.7				
25 to 49 hours	21	15.4				
less than 25 hours	33	24.3				
(Total in-home hours used: 14,507)						
75 or more days			0	—		
50 to 74 days			1	8.3		
25 to 49 days			2	16.7		
less than 25 days			9	75.0		
(Total day-care days used: 208)						
21 or more days					3	6.8
14 to 20 days					12	27.3
7 to 13 days					21	47.8
less than 7 days					8	18.1
(Total nursing home days used: 501)						

89

The 136 caregivers using in-home respite received a total of 14,507 hours of such help in the course of the year, or a mean of 107 hours. The amounts of in-home help used varied widely, however, from 24% who used less than 24 hours to 36% who used 100 or more hours during the project year (Table 4.7). There was also significant variation in the length of time the service was utilized. Ten percent of in-home service users employed it for 10 to 12 months, 11% for 7 to 9 months, 37% for 3 to 6 months, and 42% for less than 3 months during the project year.

Day Care

Four percent of the families in the experimental respite program used only day care respite provided through the FRCP program. Those 12 families used a total of 208 days, or a mean of 17 days. (It must be kept in mind, however, that a much larger number of families in the program received day care from other sources.)

Institutional Respite

Fourteen percent of the family care givers who used the experimental services chose institutional respite, all of which took place in nursing homes. Of the families who used institutional respite, 71% used it once, 27% twice, and 2% used it on more than 2 occasions. The number of days used on each occasion ranged from 3 days to 3 weeks.

Families chose the nursing-home form of respite primarily when they needed an extended period of complete relief. Approximately half of the caregivers who used such respite did so when they required surgery or had an emergency hospitalization. Others used it for vacations, to visit out of town relatives, to be at home for an uninterrupted time to relax, to spend time with children and grandchildren, to attend a religious retreat, or to plan for long-term care by going to visit nursing homes.

What can be concluded from this naturalistic experiment to test demand through the offer of assistance to a pool of caregivers is, first, that only a little over half availed themselves of the offer. Second, the most popular experimentally offered service by far was in-home respite services. Day care was also relatively frequently used but not through the experimental program. Nursing-home respite was infrequently used. A third conclusion is that the proportion of experimental respite users who paid completely or partially for the services was relatively high, 50%.

WHICH CLIENTS USED RESPITE SERVICES?

Caregivers who are most stressed and who have fewest opportunities for relief ought to be greater users. Therefore the following attributes were hypothesized to be "risk factors" associated with the need for and use of respite care services: living with the impaired person; being a spouse caregiver; older age of both impaired person and caregiver; severity of the impaired person's symptoms; degree of caregiving burden; lower physical and psychological well-being in the caregiver; less preprogram use of formal and informal services and respite in particular.

The statistical analysis was designed to show the relationships between these variables as they were measured prior to the experimental respite program for the experimental group and the actual amount of use of experimental respite: Amount of in-home respite, amount of nursing home respite, amount of day care, and total amount of respite used. Because the risk factors were related to one another, the analysis was done using multiple regression analysis, which determined effects of each risk factor independent of the effects of the other risk factors.

As a way of summarizing a complex set of findings, it is easiest to begin by noting that a number of the presumed risk factors were unrelated to the amount of respite care used. It did not seem to matter whether the caregiver lived with the impaired person or not, nor did spouses use the services more than did caregivers with different relationships to the older person. Healthy caregivers used respite to the same degree as less healthy caregivers. Even the severity of cognitive symptoms (i.e., typical symptoms of intellectual decline as seen in dementing illness) was unrelated to use of services. The amounts of help received from others by the caregiver during the twelve months before the experimental respite program began—including paid respite care, informal respite care (primarily from other family members), and other services, whether from informal or formal sources—were also unrelated. Finally, three facets of caregiving attitudes measured at baseline—social impact of caregiving, caregiving mastery, and caregiving satisfaction—were unrelated to the amount of use of any type of respite.

Looking next at the client characteristics associated with amount of respite use, it is convenient to examine each type of respite separately.

Day Care

Only one of the risk factors was related to how much day care was used; impaired people with behavioral symptoms and socially inappropriate behavior were less likely to use day care.

In-Home Respite

Caregivers of elders who showed more frequent social and behavioral symptoms were higher users of in-home respite. The strongest determinant of use of such services was a high degree of subjective caregiving burden reported by the caregiver. Only these two risk factors, out of a total of 20, showed significant (at a probability level less than .01) prediction of in-home service use.

Nursing Home Respite

This type of respite was used more frequently by older caregivers and in behalf of older impaired persons. The nursing home was also more likely to be used by caregivers who were spending more time in caregiving at the beginning of the study. It is very likely that these same families were those in which caregiving emergencies, such as sickness of the caregiver, were more frequent.

Total Amount of Respite Care Use

A somewhat more consistent effect of the risk factors was seen when all forms of respite were aggregated. Overall, more respite was used for older impaired elders, by caregivers who were more burdened by their caregiving and who devoted more time to that task. In addition, this overall analysis showed greater use by caregivers who were depressed and those who reported fewer positive emotions at baseline.

In summary, client family characteristics did predict respite use, but to a lesser extent than might have been expected. It should be noted that older impaired people and older caregivers are likely to constitute a spouse-caregiver family and therefore to share a household. Therefore, the significant effects of age for both probably includes some tendency for spouses and those sharing the household to use respite more, even though these effects were not independent of age.

The nature of the disability was associated with the type of service chosen. When behavioral problems were greater, for example, more in-home and less day care was used. It is obvious that behavioral problems are barriers to use of day care, both because of the difficulties of getting such patients ready and transporting them to the site of the service and because many day care centers exclude patients with such characteristics.

This thin list of significant relationships was overshadowed by the failure of many others that might have been expected to predict the use of respite services: Most types of caregiving attitudes, mental health indicators, and physical health were unrelated to use of services. Even more importantly, those who were relatively poorly supplied with formal or informal respite help before the intervention were no more likely to avail themselves of the offer of experimental respite than were those who already had such services in place.

In conclusion, for this caregiver group it was difficult to forecast who might use the services. Later in this volume some further suggestions regarding factors that may lead to use of respite will be discussed. They are based on qualitative case material, however. The formal quantitative risk factors were simply not very powerful predictors.

PAYMENT FOR RESPITE SERVICES

Forty percent of the families who used the FRCP subsidy also paid some of the costs themselves. Cost figures must be interpreted carefully, however, because they reflect only the actual use of the FRCP respite subsidy. Many families who used day care and in-home service used the subsidy one week and paid entirely on their own the next week. Those with more financial resources often paid for the services on their own. The overwhelming majority of families were judicious in their use of respite services.

Caregivers with the lowest incomes are overrepresented in the following statistics: Of the families who used the subsidy, 27% used less than $250, 20% used $250 to $499, 15% used $500 to $739, 39% used $750 to $1000, 75% did not go beyond an additional $200.00. In short, only about 5% of families using respite needed significantly more than the $1000 cap and the larger amounts were used when families encountered crisis situations such as hospitalization of the caregiver.

Families were not told routinely that there was a cap of $1000 on the FRCP subsidy. Rather, they were first helped to arrive at a respite plan, then offered the subsidy as needed. Some families did ask about the limitations of the subsidy and the $1000 of available assistance became part of their planning. A very few caregivers refused to consider their own resources in planning for respite and used the entire respite subsidy available to them. These were people who feared depleting their own resources so that they would not have funds for respite or long-term care institutionalization when they "really needed it."

Overall, the caregiving families were extraordinarily modest in their request for services and were willing (even eager) in most cases to pay what they could afford.

THE WAY THE FAMILIES USED
THE THREE TYPES OF RESPITE SERVICE

In-Home Respite

Most people are familiar with in-home assistance for matters unrelated to elder care such as cleaning, "baby-sitting," and nursing and medical care. It may be that in-home help in caring for an impaired older person is an understandable and natural extension of that concept. For those caregivers who had difficulty giving themselves permission to leave the patient simply to "have a good time," in-home respite was often used to do tasks necessary to managing a household such as grocery shopping.

The acceptability of in-home respite may also have been due to the fact that most of the families put the needs and feelings of the patient before their own. Therefore, it was more acceptable to have a type of respite that did not change the latter's environment. Another incentive for selecting in-home respite is that it is the most flexible of all respite services, as it can be adjusted more readily to the amounts and specific times that respite is wanted. It can, for example, be provided for long or short periods of time, at night or during the day, and on weekdays or weekends. Finally, in-home respite can be used for patients with varying degrees of impairment, levels of functioning, and differing behaviors and personalities. The impaired people in the program ranged from those in the very early stages of dementia to those who required one-to-one supervision or were bedbound.

Although in-home respite was the most frequently chosen type of respite, it does have some limitations. First, it is expensive when used for long periods of time. An eight-hour day of in-home respite costs twice as much as a day of day care, and overnight in-home respite is more costly than institutional respite care. Secondly, some families are reluctant to allow strangers into their homes. Third, homemakers/companions are often poorly trained and low paid; as a result, the reliability and quality of the service they provide is sometimes questionable. (The staff on our project worked with homemaker agencies to identify a cadre of homemakers who would receive some training about dementia and who could be counted on for reliability.) Fourth, for some families, the emotional costs to the family far exceeded the emotional benefits.

> After many months of counseling because of Mrs. H.'s initial reluctance to use respite service (her mother had taken care of her and now it was "her turn" to take care of her mother), in-home respite was scheduled for four hours monthly so that she could attend a social event. When the social worker called Mrs. H. after the first respite episode, the latter was upset because the respite worker had been late. As a result, Mrs. H. worried the entire time she was out about her mother's care. She did not want to try another homemaker because she was afraid that the first one would find out and retaliate against the family. The social worker counseled the caregiver about how the first time leaving her mother was the most difficult and that sometimes the match between homemaker and family did not work out. Mrs. H. was persuaded to try a different homemaker and this time the experience was successful.

Day Care

Among the beneficial aspects of day care is that it offers freedom from caregiving responsibilities for a relatively long, continuous block of time—generally six to eight hours. This was particularly important for caregivers who wanted to use the time to rest at home or to do household chores. The cost was also an advantage, as the same number of in-home hours of respite would have cost approximately twice as much. An excellent incentive for using day care was that it offered stimulation and socialization for the patient. Caregivers who were reluctant to use respite for their own needs were able to rationalize it as good for their patient.

An elderly, isolated caregiver, Mrs. E. suffered from multiple health problems and was exhausted from caring for her demented husband. Yet she refused respite and other types of help as she felt that her husband was her responsibility. Mrs. E. told the social worker that prior to becoming ill her husband had enjoyed getting together with friends from work. The social worker suggested that perhaps he would enjoy day care for socialization.

Reluctantly, Mrs. E. agreed to try day care for her husband's well-being. The experience was so successful that day care was increased from once weekly to three times weekly. After several months of day care, Mrs. E. confided to the social worker that she was able to do chores and sleep while her husband was at day care. She felt that the service was as good for her as it was for her husband.

For families who were burdened by taking the impaired person to numerous medical appointments, the PGC Day Care Center—which offered medical services—had the extra benefit of providing one-stop shopping.

Although separation from the patient often was difficult, caregivers felt that day care offered a supervised professional experience and were certain that their impaired relatives would be cared for well. A small number of families whose patients were in the early stages of dementia reported that day care was the only form of respite they could use. The socialization component of that service proved to be acceptable to the patients as well.

The greatest barrier to the use of day care was its lack of availability. While day care at PGC was available to project families, many lived at too great a distance to make the PGC program feasible. At the beginning of the experimental respite project, other agency subsidies for in-home and institutional respite were practically nonexistent in the Philadelphia area. During the subsequent year, however, four new day care centers opened and subsidies for day care were offered through the local Area Agency on Aging, the Philadelphia Corporation for Aging (PCA), though waiting lists were long. Nevertheless, because project staff referred caregivers for those subsidies, probably far fewer caregivers relied on the project for day care subsidies than otherwise would have.

Other factors precluded the use of day care even when it was available. Most day care centers in the Philadelphia area and elsewhere have behavioral and functional eligibility criteria. Patients with behavioral problems such as wandering and incontinence are often excluded, for example, and those in the late stages of the disease can rarely be handled in day care programs. Transportation may not be available. Too much physical and emotional effort may be required to induce an impaired member to leave the home and for the caregiver to complete the tasks involved in getting them on the bus. The hours of day care may not correspond to a family's greatest need for respite—at night or on weekends, for example. A small number of families were unable to be away from their impaired person for an entire day. Finally, some caregivers wanted to use day care respite sporadically for special events, rather than routinely, but day care as it exists in the Philadelphia area is designed for regular, rather than occasional, use.

Institutional Respite

Institutional respite has several advantages: (1) it offers extended relief at about half the cost of a comparable amount of in-home respite; (2) the nursing home is a supervised, professional setting equipped to handle emergencies, which seems to alleviate family anxiety about care; (3) nursing homes have the capability to cope with a range of patient behavioral problems or severe functional disabilities.

There were several obstacles to the use of institutional respite. Limitation on funds was the main reason families did not use it more often and for longer periods of time. The vast majority of caregivers were trying to avoid permanent institutionalization of the patient and the prospect of even a short-term nursing home placement evoked fears about this possibility. Furthermore, like the general population, the caregivers had been well-indoctrinated by the media about nursing home scandals and patient abuse. They had a range of other concerns as well: fear that their loved ones would not receive individualized attention, that they would respond poorly to a change of environment, or that they would be fearful if placed with nursing home residents who were less intact than themselves.

An additional barrier is that preparation for a nursing home stay is generally complicated and time-consuming. After securing medical information from doctors, there are many forms to be filled out, clothes and personal effects to be labeled and packed, and most importantly, explanations made to the mentally impaired person. Finally, some nursing homes set a minimum number of days that the patient can stay and the limits do not always fit the caregiver's plans.

Combinations of Respite Services

Fifteen percent of the experimental families used combinations of the different types of respite service. Most of those used nursing home respite in combination with either in-home (primarily) or day care respite. Each type of respite met different needs. For example, nursing homes were used when longer periods of relief were needed for vacations or when the caregiver needed hospitalization. Some of the handful of caregivers who combined day care and in-home respite had patients whose needs increased so that they could no longer be accommodated in day care. Others used day care regularly and requested in-home service for a special event. Only one family used all three types of respite.

Care-Sharing

Care-sharing in the sense that other family members were encouraged to give additional emotional or concrete assistance to the primary caregiver proved successful in a few cases. The small number of situations in which care-sharing increased should not be interpreted as a rationale for failing to make efforts to effect such sharing, as it was extremely valuable in those cases.

Care-sharing by caregivers from different families was a totally unsuccessful effort, however. This is foreseeable and understandable. The extraordinary difficulties of caring for an Alzheimer's patient make it unlikely that a caregiver can provide help to two such patients even for a few hours, particularly in view of the need to bring one patient to the home of another. (In that vein, a major effort at effecting such care-sharing is experiencing major problems. Stone (1986) stated that a care-sharing project in Michigan, Elder Care Share, was having difficulty recruiting families to participate.)

To summarize what was learned about service use, caregivers began by having been resourceful in their ability to use both formal and informal services. They continued this behavior during the project year. One of the goals of the experimental service, to assist caregivers in matching the entire array of possible services to their needs, was achieved and documented in the selectively greater use of some services by the experimental group. Experimental respite services were used by just over half of all families who were offered the service. To a mild extent, greater vulnerability did seem to encourage families to use respite. The case management and counseling process yielded a great deal of information on why people chose to use or not to use the services.

The Effects of
the Experimental
Respite Program

5

This chapter will describe the evaluation of the effects of respite care. The major portion will examine the effects of the experimental intervention on the impaired person and on the well-being of the caregiver. The caregiver's direct evaluation of the program was also assessed. Finally, the effects of the respite care on the volume of use of other formal services and on the amount of informal help received from the primary caregiver and others were assessed.

EFFECTS ON THE IMPAIRED PERSON

The first level of the assessment of the effect of the respite program was to determine whether differences existed between experimental and control groups in impaired-person outcomes, that is, life span and length of community tenure.

After 12 months a similar number of experimental and control subjects were still alive (81% and 79%, respectively). Also, a very slight and insignificant difference emerged when comparing the groups in terms of the percentages who remained outside an institution, which was 64% among experimentals and 59% among controls.

Considering the overall strength of the treatment (i.e., a relatively mild level of assistance, used by only half the subjects), it would be expecting a great deal to think that the prolongation of the impaired person's life could be affected. Even the prolongation of the period of community residence is a stringent expectation. Therefore, it is likely that the major impacts, if any, would be found among the indicators of social and psychological well-being that were used in this research.

Analysis of the effects of respite on outcome assumes equality of the experimental and control groups at the beginning of the study, an assumption that would be reasonable for a very large population assigned randomly to the two groups. While comfortably large by comparison with most randomized experimental studies, our sample is small by epidemiological standards. Therefore, the bare comparisons of longevity and community tenure need to be augmented by comparison methods that take into account both the baseline levels of the two groups in other variables that might be associated with outcome and the amount of time the impaired person remained in the community. The next section describes the multivariate analysis of the two impaired-persons outcomes, a survival analysis.

This better-controlled analytic model used days alive and days in community as continuous outcome variables. Before comparing experimental and control groups, baseline levels of possible risk factors were statistically accounted for, as shown in Table 5.1. The set of variables predicted survival significantly, but the difference between control and experimental groups (the first independent variable shown in Table 5.1) was not one of the significantly differentiating variables. On the other hand, when number of days in the community was used as the dependent variable—that is, time from baseline to (1) death, (2) placement in a nursing home, or (3) the full 12 months until the Time 2 evaluation for the community-alive

Table 5.1. Survival Analysis of Experimental and Control Groups: Longevity and Community Tenure[a]

Baseline independent variable (covariate)	Days alive	Days in community
Control versus experimental	1.46	2.63**
Age of caregiver	− .18	−1.17
Sex of caregiver	.87	− .51
Education of caregiver	−1.52	−2.80**
Sex of impaired person	2.87**	.52
Age of impaired person	−1.19	− .59
Racial status of impaired person	−1.60	− .24
Caregiver is spouse of older person	.40	.27
Caregiver lives with older person	.03	.51
Number of cognitive symptoms	2.82**	4.23**
Number of noncognitive symptoms	−2.13*	− .77
Informal respite, year before baseline	2.13*	2.38*
Informal secondary caregivers	2.29*	1.43
Help given by primary caregiver	.09	1.37
Formal services, year before baseline	− .47	− .34
Subjective burden	1.51	2.45*
Traditional caregiving ideology	.08	.43
Caregiving competence	− .02	1.17
Caregiving uplifts	− .04	.59
Caregiving impact	−1.17	−1.41
Log likelihood ratio	598.2	1212.2
Chi square ($df = 20$)	50.5**	55.2**

[a]Cell entries represent ratios of regression coefficients to their standard errors, distributed as z.
*$p < .05$.
**$p < .01$.

group,—not only was the whole set of predictors significantly related to community tenure, but experimental subjects remained in the community significantly longer than did control subjects ($z = 2.63$, $p < .01$). The regression coefficient associated with the experimental versus control contrast indicated that the number of days in the community was 22 days longer for the experimental group than for the control group net of the other 19 factors.

Other information portrayed in Table 5.1 shows that having had fewer symptoms and more informal respite care during the year prior to the study was associated with longer life and more days in the community. Longevity was also associated with the impaired person's being female and with more secondary informal caregivers. Longer community tenure was also associated with lower caregiver education and less expression of subjective caregiving burden at baseline.

THE SUBJECTIVE WELL-BEING OF THE CAREGIVER

The effect of respite care on subjective well-being is the most complex question to answer among those posed by the research. Regression analysis of differences in well-being at Time 2 as a function of the respite intervention was the analytic strategy, controlling for background and risk factors for 341 community-alive subjects only; none of the families in the other three groups had comparable treatment experiences or well-being outcome measures totally similar to those whose impaired person remained in the community for the whole year. Therefore, analyses dealing with caregiving appraisal could not be performed on the total group of all 632 subjects.

For four outcome variables, however, depression, negative affect, positive affect, and self-rated health of caregiver, a regression analysis of caregiver well-being based on all caregivers regardless of the status of the impaired person at Time 2 was performed.

Finally, since only about half of all caregivers in the experimental respite group availed themselves of experimental services, a series of analyses within the experimental group was performed to test the effects of actual use of the experimental services on well-being at Time 2.

Effects of 12 Months of Enrollment
in the Experimental Respite Program

At this point it is necessary to reiterate that the experimental-versus-control contrast actually represented the difference between those who were offered experimental respite and those who were not offered the service. Two factors moderate the clarity of the experimental-versus-control difference. First, not all who were offered the service used it. Second, substantial use was made of respite services by members of the control group acting on their own initiative. Nonetheless, because of the extensive program of assessment, case management, education and counseling, as well as the sense of security that there would be help available if needed, the assignment to the experimental group may be presumed to have been a positive intervention.

To test the difference between experimental and control groups on the indicators of caregiving appraisal, a series of multiple regressions was performed for the community-alive group using each of the five indices of appraisal as dependent variables: subjective caregiving burden, caregiving mastery, caregiving impact, caregiving satisfaction, and traditional caregiving ideology. The effects of background characteristics, living arrangement, symptom intensity (stressor), and amount of formal and informal respite received during the year before baseline were controlled by using measures of these attributes as independent variables in the regressions. Regressed change scores (i.e., the baseline value of the Time 2 dependent variable was used as a control variable) failed to reveal any effect of the experimental respite program on caregiving appraisal.

Selective Effects of Respite
on People with Risk Factors

One of the study's hypotheses was that families with special needs would be selectively benefited by the experimental respite program. These special needs, or risk factors, were: more frequent or intense symptoms in the impaired person, being a spouse caregiver versus other types of caregivers, being a care-giver who lived in the household with the impaired person, and families who began the research year with less formal and informal respite during the previous 12 months. The effects of the risk factors were tested by means of the statistical interaction (cross-product) between a risk factor and the experimental or control group assignment. These interaction tests asked the question, "Was the experimental program selectively more efficacious with families of deprived status in each of the risk factors?"

No significant effects were evidenced for experimental respite directed toward the originally deprived subjects.

Effects of the Experimental Program on Physical and Psychological Well-being— Risk Factors and Effects

The four ultimate outcome criteria of well-being—self-rated health, negative affect, positive affect, and depression—were assessed at baseline and the 12-month follow-up occasion for all caregivers, regardless of whether the impaired person lived for the full year, went to a nursing home, or remained in the community for the year. For these analyses, the differing length of exposure to the possibility of receiving respite was taken account of as a control variable before testing the relationship between experimental respite and regressed change scores in the four indicators of well-being.

Again, there was no independent relationship between intervention and physical or psychological outcome. Neither was any risk factor associated with differential change in well-being by these four criteria.

Effects of Use of Experimental Respite Services on Caregivers

It is worthwhile emphasizing at this point that, despite the assignment of subjects to the experimental respite group and the offer of respite services to all of these families, only 52%

actually used experimental respite services. The present section will analyze the relationship between the use of various experimental respite services and the outcomes associated with well-being: caregiver health, positive affect, negative affect, depression, in-community days and days alive.

It is important to underline the fact that the decision as to whether to use the experimental services was almost always made by the caregiver. Such self-selection means that any relationships observed between service use and outcomes are ambiguous in causal direction. That is, it is possible that the use of a service might have an effect on an indicator of well-being. However, the interpretation that lower well-being might be the cause of a service's being chosen is equally plausible.

Within the experimental group, regression analyses were done for the 171 community-alive experimental families and the total of 262 experimental families (for the four ultimate health-outcome well-being criteria), using the summed amount of experimental respite as the focal predictor. Amount of experimental respite did not affect any of the outcomes, nor did the addition of a variable representing the amount of respite received over and above the amount of experimental respite received increase prediction of favorable change in well-being. Finally, risk factors were again irrelevant to outcome.

To summarize this section of the assessment of experimental effect, there was no evidence at all that either experimental respite or respite procured by the family on its own affected either caregiver-specific well-being (the five facets of caregiving appraisal) or the more general indicators of physical and mental health. Neither was there any ability of experimental respite to show particular efficacy when applied to people with special deprivations or original stress.

CAREGIVERS' EVALUATIONS OF RESPITE CARE

An important indicator of the success of any service is the caregiver's evaluation of the quality of the respite received and the impact of the respite on his or her daily life.

Before presenting the results regarding such an evaluation it is worthwhile relating this phase of the inquiry to a theoretical framework espoused by one of us (Lawton, 1983) regarding a concept of "the good life." An argument was made that all that was desirable as a personal or social goal could be subsumed in four sectors of the good life: psychological well-being, behavioral competence, the objective environment, and perceived quality of life. The assertion was made that while well-being in one sector is often correlated with well-being in another sector, the values and norms defining goodness or desirability in any sector *may* be independent of definitions of goodness in another. Yet as individuals and as societies, people strive for the satisfaction inherent in very limited domains of any of these sectors. Therefore, such goals can be construed as having intrinsic value in their own right, rather than depending for their social value on their ability to elevate well-being in some other sector.

In the respite research, one of many domains of our caregivers' lives is the limited area of giving care to the impaired elder. One could say that a subdomain of behavioral competence is the skill exercised in giving such care. One's feelings of satisfaction as a caregiver and one's feelings (whether positive or negative) about the quality of the way one's time is spent thus constitute a limited but important component of the caregiver's total way of life. It seems just as important to ask the person what having respite did for the quality of daily life and their overt evaluation of what was provided, as to ask whether the caregiver's level of depression changed after respite was offered. This section will deal with a set of such directly evaluative questions. Some of the results may be directly useful in the tailoring of new respite services to people's needs.

EVALUATIONS OF GENERIC RESPITE SERVICES

Because many people in the control group had respite services and others in the experimental group did not use such services, an attempt was made to inquire about achieved respite in generic terms that would be applicable to either people who were experimental respite clients or those who were not.

One question relevant to the usefulness of respite care to the caregiver is the use to which time freed from caregiving duties by respite is put. The background against which respite care occurs was an average of about 8.4 hours per day spent in caregiving activities. Therefore we asked the 92% of the experimental group and the 85% of the control group who reported having some form of respite care how they spent the extra time afforded by the respite. About 40% overall stated unequivocally that they used the time totally for themselves, while all but about a residual 10% indicated that they spent such time in different mixes of self- and other-directed activity.

Subjects were asked to rate how relieved they were by having respite care, how much the older person liked the respite care, and how satisfied they were, overall, with the respite they received. The plurality of all ratings was strongly on the positively evaluative side. Among those whose older person remained in the community, 72% of the experimental caregivers were "greatly" or "very greatly" relieved by respite, as compared to 59% of the controls. Similar percentages were 77% for experimentals and 64% for controls in being "very satisfied" with respite care. Both differences were statistically significant, reflecting the higher evaluation by the group exposed to experimental respite.

Caregivers' judgments as to how the impaired person seemed to assess the respite program were, not surprisingly, less favorable. Forty-four percent of caregivers in the experimental group said their impaired relative liked respite "a lot" or "a little," as opposed to 51% in the control group (difference not significant). This finding should be used in the training of respite workers, sensitizing them to the impaired person's probable feelings of strangeness and possible rejection of people other than familiar caregivers.

Three open-ended questions, with no reference to the experimental respite program, respite services in other forms, or any specific service, were asked regarding the caregiver's experience with services over the past year. The questions asked were:

1. What kinds of help that others gave, or services you received this past year, were most helpful to you and (elder) in his/her care? (see responses in Table 5.2)
2. Were there any problems with the help or services you received last year?
3. What (more) would you have liked in the way of assistance with your caregiving?

Three or four responses to each question were accepted and coded into a 96-item category code of the most specific kinds of assistance that could be coded. The major specific categories were then collapsed into the smaller number of service categories shown in Table 5.2, using the system indicated in the footnote to the table.

These questions were not asked at all in a context that might selectively elicit respite-related responses. Yet as Table 5.2 shows, by far the most helpful types of services were those classified as respite. Of even greater interest is that this pattern was equally true for the experimental and control groups. After respite, the in-home personal care and instrumental or health assistance services ran far ahead of any others. The only category in which the experimental and control difference is really noteworthy is in the nursing-home respite category, where the experimental group was the only one to have experienced this type of respite to any significant degree.

Table 5.2 indicates that very few people in either the experimental or the control group felt that any service was problematic. However, the great preponderance of such problems were found specifically in services delivered by home-health aides. This kind of unskilled assistance has long been known to be problematic. These data point once more to the need for upgrading training efforts among such staff.

The services wished for more often show a similar pattern to that of the most-helpful services, with respite the major

Table 5.2. Service Evaluation During the Research Year

Service	Most helpful		Problematic		Wished more often	
	E	C	E	C	E	C
None named	18	22	187	162	64	38
Health	24	34	5	11	12	12
Personal care	70	69	8	4	54	34
In-home IADL/health	85	90	46	32	51	48
Respite						
institutional	26	4	7	0	3	6
day care	55	49	4	6	14	16
in-home, other	110	149	12	6	100	120
Counseling	14	6	0	0	3	12
Support	28	38	0	1	18	21
Socialization	4	22	0	0	5	6
Transportation	18	16	3	7	8	5
Financial	8	3	1	0	13	9
Educational	3	1	0	0	1	2
Other	7	7	2	2	33	25
Number of responses	452	487	88	69	316	316
Number of subjects	290	268				

Subjects could name up to 4 services in response to each open-ended question. Health: Doctor, in-home medical, hospital, therapy; in-home: IADL assistance, meals, home health aide; respite other: paid, unpaid, in or out of home; support: support groups, emotional support; socialization: visitors, recreation, senior center.

wished-for category and the in-home cluster the second. One interesting experimental-versus-control difference is seen in the greater tendency for experimental subjects to report having wished for no additional services—another indicator that the experimental respite program met some people's needs very exactly.

The only outcome group with an opportunity to use such services in the future (the community-alive group) was asked to estimate plans for use of respite services in the coming year. About three-quarters of all people planned to use some form of service, and their ordering roughly paralleled the "most helpful" and "wished more" columns of Table 5.2. Unpaid sitters

(49%) and paid sitters at home (52%) were the most likely to be planned. Day care would be likely for 38% and nursing-home respite for 18%, both of the latter slightly more likely for the experimental group that had been offered these services.

In summary, this open-ended effort to evaluate services delivered ended up with the most striking affirmation of the perceived value of respite services: Those services given were very highly regarded but the need was by no means met. It is very likely also that the ordinary in-home services that were both liked and wished for also served some respite needs as well. The big problems are (a) getting enough such time, and (b) elevating the quality of such services. Those services that used paid outsiders were seen as most problematic.

The last component of the direct-evaluation section focused on the experimental respite as an object. Caregivers in the experimental group were asked a series of questions regarding the experimental program in the format, "Did you receive help with ____?," regarding a series of caregiving problems. If the answer was "yes," the subject rated "how much" help was received and how satisfied they were with that aspect of the help.

The results for the combined groups are shown in Table 5.3. It must be remembered that every experimental subject received an extensive initial assessment and discussion of their personal situation and an at-least basic amount of case management time throughout the year, initiated by the experimental respite project worker if the caregiver family did not contact the service on her own. However, personal counseling, family counseling, and educational activity among other services were provided only selectively. A given family would be expected to have discussed only a few of all possible issues or to have received help in only selected areas. For example, many families never experienced anything that they construed as "a crisis." Therefore, many would not have received any assistance "during a caregiving crisis." Another example is "ask family for respite"—the great majority were already receiving such family assistance and so the question was irrelevant to the majority.

Table 5.3. Types of Help Received and Satisfaction with Help Experimental Respite Subjects

Type of help	Percentage of received help[a]	Percentage very satisfied[b]
Overall help	85.8	78.9
Information on respite	57.2	69.7
Help figuring respite needs	67.9	74.2
Information on finding respite services	70.2	67.8
Ideas on how to ask family for respite	36.3	65.3
Information on how to arrange respite	67.8	64.6
Help paying for respite	53.6	89.0
Encouragement to use respite	84.9	73.4
Help planning for future respite	46.1[c]	71.4[c]
Emotional support	80.8	79.4
Ideas on how to cope with caregiving	57.7	70.2
Help during a caregiving crisis	33.5	68.2
Information on medical services	35.9	69.6
Information on support groups	56.6	58.1
Information on legal services	21.9	61.7
Information on entitlements	17.7	56.6

[a]Percentage indicating "much" or "some" help received.
[b]Percentage "very satisafied," of all receiving that form of help.
[c]Percentages calculated only for Community Alive group ($N = 174$).

In any case, inspection of Table 5.3 shows that two classes of help stand out as having been received most widely: first, assistance with information on or arranging for respite care, and second, emotional support. Those types of assistance for which least help was perceived as having been given, in addition to those mentioned above, were related to nonrespite issues such as legal and entitlement questions, and to assistance implying substantial caregiver problems ("cope with caregiving"). In addition, fewer than half received financial assistance, and a greater proportion indicated that they received no assistance in finding support groups; however, it is likely that these represented families already connected with such groups (about one-third of all caregiver families). Although it is not possible to partition the "none received" category into those who would have liked help and those who did not need or wish help, the high levels of satisfaction expressed by those who received every kind of assistance make it seem likely that a good match between need and type of help received was attained.

Satisfaction was least felt in getting information on support groups. Clinical reports indicate that the location of a support group near their dwelling was a very important feature of the group for caregivers and many could not find one that met this locational criterion. Thus, it is useful for planning purposes to recognize this potential area for improvement—in developing more groups, disseminating information about them, and helping caregivers to access them.

In summary, the consumer-survey type of information portrayed in Table 5.3 attests to the positive regard in which the experimental respite program was held, very close to 80% being very satisfied.

THE EFFECT OF EXPERIMENTAL RESPITE ON OTHER SERVICES

The last two research questions regarding the effects of experimental respite are different from the others discussed previously in this chapter. The earlier questions concerned effects on various facets of family well-being. Those to be discussed next concern the relationships among different aspects of the total service context.

The various services, respite or others, the formal and informal services given, and the specific help given by the primary caregiver may be looked upon as a system of mutually dependent activities conducted in the interest of serving the needs of an impaired older person. If need is constant, then a change in one type of service provision would be likely to cause other service provisions to be rearranged. A frequent situation exists in which need is high but the service context does not provide enough volume of services, or the right mix, to serve the need. In this case an augmentation of one type of service might have no effect on the others already in place. Yet another scenario might cause the increase in use of one type of service to "liberate" some latent demand for other types of services; the liberation effect could happen either with no change in original level of need or in response to increased need.

Two questions were asked in their part of the research.

1. Does the case-management process associated with offering respite care affect the provision of other formal services?

This first question is relevant for service planning. Given the structure for offering respite services, can the service agency expect the case-management process to promote the use of additional services beyond those that are explicitly for respite purposes?

2. Does the provision of formal respite care services lead to service substitution; that is, is there a reduction in existing informal services, either respite or nonrespite services, following the offering of the experimental respite?

The issue of whether providing formal services substitutes for the efforts of family, friends, and others is an old issue in the social services arena. In general, in other contexts the evidence has failed to document major substitution (Kemper et al., 1986; Zimmer & Mellor, 1981). Despite the general failure to document the service substitution phenomenon, it seems desirable to test this possibility with respect to every new type of service or manner of delivering the service.

Effect of the Experimental Respite Program on the Receipt of All Formal Services

Table 5.4 shows the mean number of units of each of 13 formal services received during the year before baseline and during the treatment year for the 345 community-alive subjects who had the full year's opportunity to use the services. The distribution of these services was very skewed. As was shown in Table 4.5, most services were not used at all by the

Table 5.4. Mean Number of Formal Service Units Per Year, Baseline and Time 2 Community Alive Group

Service	Control		Experimental	
	BL	T2	BL	T2
Homemaker visits	15.9	20.5	9.4	22.0
Home-delivered meals (days)	6.2	7.9	7.8	11.0
Home-health aide/personal care visits	22.7	41.6	30.6	50.0
Visiting nurse visits	3.5	6.1	6.4	7.2
Therapeutic visits (OT, PT, other) visits	2.4	.8	2.0	1.5
Transportation (one-way trips)	32.1	53.6	24.8	48.1
Shopping trips	.4	.6	.4	.9
In-home respite hours	337.0	412.1	137.3	379.5
Physician visits	10.5	10.3	11.7	16.3
Psychiatric hospital days	1.2	.8	1.7	.8
Acute hospital days	8.7	6.8	5.6	6.1
Nursing home days	.8	2.0	.4	2.4
Day care hours	103.8	153.3	64.8	229.0

majority of the families. Despite such distributional differences among services, the total pattern shown by the means is very coherent.

The entire array of baseline to Time 2 service use estimates for experimental and control subjects across the 13 services was subjected to a multivariate analysis of variance (MANOVA), a method of testing experimental versus control group differences that takes account of the correlations among the types of service use. The data were transformed logarithmically to compensate for the skew. This approach allowed the effects of the experimental versus control difference, the difference between baseline and Time 2, and the differential change from baseline to Time 2, depending on whether the family was in the experimental or the control group, to be analyzed independently of one another.

An increase in overall amount of service use from baseline to Time 2 was clearly significant (Wilks $\lambda = .776$, $F = 7.33$, 13 and 330 $d.f.$, $p < .001$). With the overall change thus having been shown to be significant, the separate tests for each service type indicated significant increases in amounts of homemaker, home health/ADL assistance, transportation, paid respite, nursing-home respite, and day care. The import of this analysis by time is that the direction of patient change is downhill and more services became necessary over the treatment year, irrespective of whether subjects were in the experimental or the control group.

Considering only the difference between the experimental and the control groups (that is, disregarding whether service use was measured at baseline or at Time 2), this comparison was not significant by multivariate test (Wilks $\lambda = .969$, $F = 0.82$, 13 and 330 $d.f.$, n.s.).

The critical test of whether the experimental group increased service use over time more than did the control group was performed by the interaction between experimental versus control and baseline versus Time 2. This test was significant (Wilks $\lambda - .921$, $F = 2.18$, 13 and 330 $d.f.$, $p < .01$). Despite the significance of the multivariate test, only one service—day care—showed a significant univariate differential increase in the experimental group. This set of findings confirms what can be seen by inspecting the changes in means of Table 5.4 from baseline to Time 2 for experimental and control groups successively across all services: There were small differential increases in the experimental group which, when all services are considered together, were significantly large. The absolute amount of increase, on the other hand, was relatively small.

Substitution of Formal Services for Informal Services

Having seen that there was a small but measurably greater increase in formal services over time for the experimental group as contrasted with the control group, the next relevant question is whether this increase was at the expense of the

informal supports that had been in place when the study
began. The major test of this question was performed by examining the volume of services performed by the primary caregiver from baseline to Time 2. If the amount of caregiving by
the primary caregiver in both experimental and control groups
diminished (given the increase in formal assistance documented in the section above), this would constitute some evidence that substitution occurred in both groups. If the assistance given by experimental group primary caregivers diminished significantly relative to change in assistance given by
control group caregivers, this would be evidence in favor of
selective service substitution within the experimental respite
group. Such a finding would suggest a hydraulic effect within
the experimental group whereby more formal services led to
fewer informal services.

Table 5.5 shows the comparative mean scores for 9 types of
assistance given by the primary caregivers of the community-
alive group at baseline and Time 2. A MANOVA test (with data
transformation) on these comparisons showed a significant
pattern of effects from baseline to Time 2; the univariate tests
indicate a decrease in banking assistance and increases in

**Table 5.5. Mean Number of Units per Year of Assistance by Primary
Caregiver, Baseline and Time 2 Community Alive Group**

Type of assistance	Control		Experimental	
	BL	T2	BL	T2
Transportation (one-way trips)	126.1	127.1	100.3	106.9
Banking	72.5	65.1	59.6	49.0
Feeding	496.4	529.8	554.6	515.2
Dressing	431.0	437.5	402.5	456.5
Grooming	280.2	323.8	254.5	265.2
Toileting	680.2	733.8	595.8	718.1
Ambulation	597.8	816.6	448.0	548.7
Bathing	173.7	219.7	195.5	215.7
Medications	705.2	636.7	686.7	715.4

toileting and ambulation assistance. There were no significant effects for the experimental versus control comparison or for the interaction. Thus there was no selective pattern of change in informal services in the experimental as compared to the control group.

Similar questions may be asked about the primary caregiver's backup services, the informal respite and personal-care assistance given by other caregivers. Table 5.6 shows the baseline and treatment-year means for experimental and control groups. The indices of number of hours per year of respite and personal-care assistance at baseline and Time 2 were transformed and analyzed by MANOVA. The experimental versus control comparison was significant (Wilks $\lambda = .965$, $F = 6.08$, $d.f. = 2,339$, $p < .01$), with the difference lying primarily in the control group's having more informal respite than did the experimental. There was no significant change (irrespective of experimental or control status) from base line to Time 2, but the significant interaction (Wilks $\lambda = .969$, $F = 5.48$, $d.f. = 2,339$, $p < .01$) indicated that the experimental group increased in amount of informal assistance proportionately more than did the control groups (by univariate test, this was significant only for personal-care assistance).

THE IMPACT OF RESPITE CARE ON THE CAREGIVER'S QUALITY OF LIFE

The theory behind respite services suggested that unrelenting caregiving demands may have unfavorable outcomes for the caregiver and the impaired person. Periodic relief of such external stress is seen, therefore, as directly therapeutic for the caregiver and indirectly for the patient.

The results of this study may be examined in terms of a series of levels that vary in degree of relevance to the respite intervention. The psychological state of the impaired person is perhaps the level most distant from the respite received by the caregiver and thus the least likely to be affected. The results from the respite evaluation showed that the respite had no

Table 5.6. Number of Hours of Informal Assistance, Baseline and Time 2: Community-Alive Group, for Control and Experimental Groups

| | Baseline | | | | | |
| | Control group | | | Experimental group | | |
Informal assistance	N	Md	X̄(all Ss)	N	Md	X̄(all Ss)
Personal-care hours	124	152	349.3	99	135	278.5
Respite hours	135	265	599.7	111	142	355.0
			Time 2			
Personal-care hours	105	156	334.2	110	222	293.7
Respite hours	135	220	675.5	114	246	466.6
Number of subjects		173			177	

meaningful measured effect on the psychological state of the impaired person.

The next level closer to the intervention itself relates the strain experienced by caregivers directly to their willingness to maintain the impaired person in the community. The results from the respite evaluation give some support to the idea that such assistance for the caregiver had favorable outcomes for the impaired person: the significantly longer period of community residence for the experimental group. The amount of gain, however—22 days as estimated by the data—is a relatively short period of time.

A level closer to the intervention is the subjective well-being of the caregiver. Indeed, enhancing caregiver well-being was the central focus of the program. Even though the precedent in the literature for expecting the intervention to improve caregiver well-being was relatively small, it is still necessary to consider carefully possible explanations for the total lack of impact of either the experimental program or actual amount of respite received on the appraised burden, physical health, or mental health of the caregiver, and the lack of such an effect even among the caregivers who were originally most stressed or most disadvantaged. The two most relevant pieces of information in this regard are, first, that by no means does every caregiver need additional respite services and, second, that the magnitude of the presumed intervention needs to be considered.

A minority of caregivers were without respite resources at the beginning of the study. Even with the ease of obtaining new respite provided by the experimental program, only half actually used these additional resources. One conclusion is that a step in planning an effective new respite service is to define a high-need group and make specific marketing appeals to this group. This project failed to show any difference in responsiveness to respite services among those who would seem to have high need: older caregivers, members of the impaired person's household, spouse caregivers, those caring for more symptomatic impaired people, or those with low base rates of respite care. Whether high need was not defined accurately or whether the respite was simply ineffective is a question that needs to be pursued in later research. More information is necessary on how caregivers who actively seek out formal respite services may differ from caregivers in general. Conceivably, some threshold level of very high need that was exceeded by few of the participants may be required for the respite intervention to have affected caregivers' subjective well-being.

It is reasonable to feel that an intervention has a greater chance for impact if it is applied more frequently, for a longer period of time (those two facets representing intensity of treatment), and with a focus on a specific problem. In the case of the experimental respite program, the intensity of project-provided services was, on the average, relatively low: among 134 users of in-home respite, the median hours used during the year was 63; among 11 users of day care the median annual days used was 19; and among 43 users of nursing-home respite the median number of days used was 11. Although the focus of respite was on affording caregivers time off, the reasons for needing the time off were so diverse that a focus on a specific problem can hardly be said to have existed. In addition, the magnitude of the intervention was limited by the fact that caregivers needed considerable time, education, and encouragement to begin to understand and use respite. They often waited until late in the caregiving process or when crises occurred to seek help.

Finally, the indicator of impact most proximate to the actual intervention of all the outcome measures was a set of questions that asked the caregivers to evaluate the service directly. Feelings of satisfaction as a caregiver and feelings (whether positive or negative) about the quality of the way time is spent constitute a limited, but important component of the caregiver's total way of life. Thus, a series of questions was used to ask the person about what having respite did for the quality of daily life and their overt evaluation of what was provided.

The evaluation given to respite service by its recipients was a resounding endorsement. Caregivers had received relief and were satisfied with the service. The service provided substitute helpers when the caregivers themselves were ill or hospitalized, allowed them to go to family events, permitted them a few hours in which to rest or catch up on household or shopping chores, and even simply enabled them to get out of the house for a short time. The results seem very clearly in support of the elevation of the quality of some hours and days in the lives of most experimental respite care users by the intervention.

THE IMPACT OF RESPITE CARE ON THE BROADER SERVICE CONTEXT

Offering Respite Care Raised Demand for Other Services Only Slightly.

During the project year, both the experimental and control-group families increased their use of formal services of various types, undoubtedly because of the inevitable downward trajectory in the functional capacities of Alzheimer's patients. Thus, both need and use increased in concert. The clear implication is that all types of respite should be available to be used flexibly. The increase in the use of other community services by the experimental group more than the controls in the course of the treatment year, although it was a very small increase, reflects one of the goals of the case-management aspect of the project. In fact, the only formal service that increased in the experimental group on its own by univariate analysis was day care, one of the targeted respite services. The selective small increase in use of other services by experimental group subjects is appropriate if we consider the respite program to have been a facilitator designed to bring service use up from a baseline of underuse and, therefore, latent need.

Thus, neither did the offer of facilitated respite services nor the assistance in procuring other services open the floodgates for an unmanageable level of demand.

Increased Formal Services
Did Not Decrease Informal Services

Additional respite and other services received by the experimental group did not encourage caregivers to reduce or withdraw their own services. In fact, caregivers in both the experimental and control groups increased the amount of help they provided during the year in which they were studied. Once more, the passage of a year in the life of severely impaired people almost certainly brought with it an increase in need. An even more noteworthy pattern was evident with secondary family caregivers. Secondary helpers were not only steadfast in the amount of help they provided, but there was actually an increase, relative to the control group, in the amount of assistance with activities of daily living provided by these other caregivers—conceivably the result of help from the experimental project staff in encouraging caregivers to find effective ways of promoting help from other family members.

Planning Respite
Programs

6

Available reports about existing respite programs often have common themes about the issues and problems with which they were confronted. Based on those reports and on the research described in this book, this chapter will identify some principles to guide professionals who wish to develop and operate respite programs.

The focus here will be on common themes and principles because there can be no one model that determines what all such programs should be like. It is generally agreed that the most desirable plan would be to include all three of the main types of respite in a comprehensive continuum of long-term care services that serves people with all types and levels of disability. The state of the art at present is, of course, far short of that ideal. There are also administrative and fiscal advantages for existing service agencies to provide respite rather than for new agencies to develop freestanding programs. However, as of 1989 there appears to be a growing number of proprietary freestanding respite services, as well as the potentially influential group of freestanding respite agencies affiliated with the Alzheimer's Association in the Robert Wood Johnson demonstration.

The relative merits of the multiservice versus freestanding model should become clear over the next few years. It is safe to anticipate, however, that various sponsors will continue to develop respite programs that depart from the ideal by, for example, offering only one or two forms of respite or respite programs that are independent of more comprehensive agencies. It is essential that those kinds of programs have firm linkages to agencies providing other long-term care services.

Programs will continue to vary in their definitions of respite, the nature of the sponsoring auspices, sources of funding, sites at which the programs take place, and in their eligibility criteria. Moreover, the programs may take place in different geographical areas and in urban, suburban, or rural environments. All of those factors play roles in determining the particular service model to be developed, including specifics such as staffing patterns, space, and equipment. If a program is to be successful in meeting the needs of the older people and families it aims to serve, these matters require the most careful advance thinking and planning.

Though the activities detailed below will be placed in a rough sequential order, the actual process cannot be expected to be orderly in that it will proceed step by step. Rather, various phases of development may be concurrent and overlapping.

Is There a Need For the Respite Program?

Among the questions to be considered early in the planning process are the type(s) of respite to be offered and the nature of the populations(s) to be served. At this writing, development of long-term care programs is uneven in that it varies not only from region to region and state to state, but even from community to community. It is vitally important to know the characteristics of the particular community in which the respite program is to take place. Information must be available about long-term care services that exist locally and about gaps in the service system. In particular, other existing respite programs, if any, should be identified.

If the program is to serve caregivers of older people with Alzheimer's disease, are data available about the number of such people in the community? Can estimates be made of the proportion of their caregivers who would use respite and the kinds of respite service those caregivers would prefer? (See Chapter 4 for data on the service yield in the PGC program.)

If Alzheimer's patients are to be the target population, can the program envisioned by the planners serve those in all stages of the disease? The type(s) of respite offered and the nature of the population serviced are interrelated. Social day care, for example, that does not include medical or nursing support can accommodate only mildly impaired patients (Quinn & Crabtree, 1987). Those who are incontinent, whose behavior is significantly disordered, or who have such major functional deficits that they need to be toileted and fed could not be cared for without explicit planning for staff sufficient to perform such services.

If the planners have the freedom to do so, they can begin from the opposite perspective. They may make an *a priori* decision, for example, that they wish to serve only care-givers who are experiencing the most strain, and choose the form(s) of respite accordingly. Because such caregivers most often have patients who are severely disabled, even bedfast, an in-home or institutional program may, therefore, be indicated.

Concurrently with the determination of care-recipient characteristics is examination of the characteristics (and needs) of the caregivers to be served. Their age, employment status, and health status are among the key characteristics that predict types and amounts of respite services that may be needed. Younger working caregivers, for example, may desire sporadic evening in-home respite services so that the family can go out, and may also desire institutional respite for family vacations. Older caregivers may require more routinely scheduled weekly respite to allow them to accomplish household tasks, keep appointments with their doctors, and have a break from the physical demands of caregiving.

Among other planning decisions that flow from the determination of who is to be served and the kind of respite service to be offered are staffing requirements, staff training, site selection, and eligibility criteria. Not least, the service context in which respite is to be embedded must be thought through.

The planning process will be enhanced by including input from consumers, or potential consumers as they are the ones with the most intimate knowledge about their needs. They can provide valuable information about all aspects of the program under consideration, particularly about defining the procedures for securing and using the service. In addition, consumers can be helpful in identifying the outreach and marketing strategies to be used.

Designing the Program

Because respite is a relatively new concept, it cannot be assumed that members of a planning group share a common understanding of what they hope to accomplish. Very early in the planning process, therefore, the planners must reach consensus about the characteristics of the population to be served, the definition of respite, and their understanding of the goals of the program they are designing. As stated in Chapter 1, respite is generally thought of as any service or group of services that provides temporary relief or rest for caregivers away from the patient. Given acceptance of such a definition, its various elements should be spelled out. What service or group of services should be offered? The main forms of respite are in-home care, institutional care, and day care, and a program can offer one or more. How is "temporary" to be interpreted? Temporary can mean in-home care either for a specified length of time, for example, or for a specified number of hours weekly on an ongoing basis. Or, it can be geared to emergency situations. Similarly, time limits can be set for the duration of institutional placement and for the number of such placements in the course of a year. Day care, too, can have time limits—for the number of days of service or for the number of times weekly, for example.

Linkages

There is a good deal of preliminary work to do in the community if the planned program is to work effectively. Because clients almost invariably need other services as well as respite, close linkages must be established with other components of the long term care system and the short-term system (e.g., acute care hospitals and step-down services) as well. The mental health system should not be overlooked in this connection. The legal system requires particular attention. Caregivers are frequently concerned about issues such as guardianship, power of attorney, living wills, and legal financial matters. Knowledgeable and willing attorneys should be identified with emphasis on locating attorneys able to serve low- and moderate-income families. (Chapter 2 listed some of the services to which the PGC respite clients were referred.) The respite program will not only be making frequent referrals to all of those agencies and professionals, but will also depend on them to make referrals to respite. The adage accepted for all planning efforts must be observed: all agencies that will be needed to implement the solution (i.e., the desired goal) must be involved at the outset.

During the planning stage, the planners, therefore, should embark on a comprehensive process of communicating with other service agencies, eliciting their views, educating them about what the respite program hopes to accomplish, and developing referral procedures. Such procedures should be streamlined— designed to facilitate linkage and to eliminate barriers to access. Overall, good relationships should be established that will ensure smooth operation of the program, with cooperation and collaboration among the agencies concerned.

Turf problems among agencies must be ironed out. A good example of such jurisdictional problems is client assessment. Even when each agency requires assessment of the caregiver/care recipient before proceeding to service provision, key assessment components should not be duplicated. Where possible, the assessment process or instrument of one agency may be able to serve as the assessment for another agency. This may require an agreement to expand the assessment areas covered by each agency. Where agencies have different foci, and the assessment process is more dissimilar than similar, parts of the assessment may be shared among agencies to avoid the necessity for caregivers to provide the same information more than once.

Another example relates to case management. Many agencies provide case management and consider it key to their service provision. When two agencies, each of which provide case management (i.e., respite program and a long-term care program) are involved with the same family, their respective roles in case management require negotiation and agreement.

The key elements in a respite program—counseling, case management, and education—were described in Chapter 2. Not all respite programs will have the capability to provide all those critical services, however, and the source of their provision must be clear at the outset. A freestanding respite program, for example, may need to rely on another organization for the counseling component, necessitating careful integration of the services.

Even agencies that will not be directly involved in the respite and care services will be in strategic positions to make referrals. Those community agencies, no less than the community at large and the potential service recipients themselves, must be educated about respite. Special attention should be paid in this regard to other health and social service agencies, local Alzheimer's Associations, Area Agencies on Aging, diagnostic units, and hospitals. Educational programs will help them to identify and refer caregivers and to create a climate of acceptance of respite.

A Family Focus

There is a basic philosophical element implicit in the definition of respite. For many years, the focus of services for the aged has been the older people themselves. Caregivers were in the background; their needs were largely ignored and they were regarded simply as providers of care to the elderly clients being served by the agency. More recently, as the negative impact of care provision on the caregivers was being documented, they have emerged from that background role so that their own needs are being recognized and legitimated. The phrase "relief or rest for caregivers" identifies the caregiver as the client. It is accepted as a given, however, that the patient's well-being must be considered. Apart from the value involved, it hardly needs repetition that the well-being of caregiver and patient are interlocked. Most caregivers are deeply concerned about the effect of their absence on their patients and the quality of the care the older people will receive in the respite situation. To underline—respite services must have a family focus that addresses the needs of both caregiver and care-recipient.

Professionals are thus confronted with the need to effect a holistic approach to the family—to strike a delicate balance so that the needs of caregiver and care-recipient are met without disadvantaging one or the other. It follows that close attention must be paid to the nature and quality of the care the older people receive.

Identifying family as well as older people as the client raises another important issue: When financial participation is indicated, whose resources should be used, the older person's or the caregiver's? Traditionally, service agencies involved in child care, for example, have used the family income to determine financial participation on a sliding scale. It would be inappropriate to use the same procedure used for elder care for services to a minor who is clearly the financial responsibility of the parents concerned.

Once decisions are reached about who pays for care and the method of determining the amounts, a method for paying the family share needs to be defined in a manner that does not create an additional burden for the caregiver. For example, caregivers of limited financial means who are paying only a portion of the costs should not be responsible for the entire costs until reimbursement is made. Billing must be simple and straightforward so as not to burden caregivers. Other "traditional" procedures also require face-to-face examination to determine whether the services offered are applicable to family care of older people. The usual practice of requiring the client to come to the agency office to apply for service may impose hardships on those providing elder care. The very nature of their need for respite—the inability to leave the patient—may preclude such a requirement.

Staffing

There is consensus that professional leadership and supervision is a *sine qua non* for respite programs of all types. Because of the nature of the services that we recommend as an integral part of any respite program, professional social workers are needed to provide the counseling and case management. It is reiterated that other staffing requirements for the respite program flow directly from the characteristics of the care recipients. Despite the successful use of volunteers in the Brookdale model (Quinn & Crabtree, 1987) and in a growing number of small volunteer-staffed programs throughout the country, many reports of respite programs have been candid in stating that volunteers cannot and do not wish to do personal care tasks for the disabled elderly. It is useful to make a careful inventory of the actual kinds of assistance the older people will need so that those needs can be matched with appropriate types of personnel. Similarly, if programming for the social and recreational needs of the older people is to take place, appropriate personnel should be included in the projected staffing pattern.

An important staffing consideration is the kind of knowledge needed by professional staff. As discussed earlier, to be effective staff must be knowledgeable about and skillful in working with older people and their families so that they can provide assessment, education, case management, and counseling. They need to be sophisticated about the health and social service system in order to access appropriate services and to advocate or negotiate for their clients. Just as important, however, is their need for extensive current knowledge about the other diverse services and resources that families frequently require. Such resources and services include barbers and beauticians who come into the home, stores in which the least expensive diapers and other supplies can be purchased, and grocery stores that deliver to the home.

Planning for appropriate staffing, does not, of course, ensure that such staff will be readily available. Provider agencies are seriously concerned about the current and future availability of personnel. The recruitment of people to provide the direct care of disabled older people is a major and critical issue. Decent wages are fundamental in attracting such workers who then must be trained to understand Alzheimer's patients and be skilled in their care.

The need for education and training extends to caregivers as well, who often are at a loss in management of behavioral problems as well as the technical aspects of care. In particular, families need to know how to prepare their patients (and themselves) for the respite experience.

An essential task of planning respite programs is the development of an outreach and marketing plan to ensure that information reaches the population the program is designed to serve. Outreach/marketing strategies will vary depending on the target population chosen, the existence and strength of community formal and informal health and social service networks, and the level of knowledge about respite in the particular community. At a minimum, each program must reach the formal (long-term care agencies, family service agencies, medical facilities) and informal (churches and synagogues, support groups) systems. As is the case with all new social service programs, visits by program staff and in-person discussions with agencies, key community leaders, and community groups yield better results than do mailings and general announcements. This is a particularly effective strategy for reaching caregivers who would not respond to general information but require help from others to encourage them to pursue respite assistance.

Program Evaluation

No respite planning process is complete without building in an evaluation component to determine whether program goals are being met. Decisions about the type of evaluation to use will reflect the financial and personnel resources available. Certain basic data are, of course, essential, such as the number of people being served, their characteristics, the amount and kinds of respite being used, referral sources, and so on. It is most important to assess caregiver satisfaction with the service. Evaluation must be specific enough to produce information that can be used to improve programs—such as consumer evaluation of specific positive and negative aspects of the service, any problems in gaining access to it, and procedural issues.

Finally, though it is a relatively recent concept, respite is quickly establishing a firm position as an essential part of the long-term care continuum. Though there is much to be learned, a substantial body of useful how-to literature is being produced, usually by centers in which early demonstrations have been performed: the New York State program (Meltzer, 1982), the Duke University program (Gwyther & Ballard, 1988; 1988), and the Brookdale program (Quinn & Crabtree, 1987). The Alzheimer's Association will continue to be a source of information on respite programming as the rapidly growing service literature accumulates.

Summary and Conclusions

7

The widespread interest in respite care has an importance that goes far beyond that particular form of help. Respite service symbolizes the growing recognition that family members caring for the disabled elderly are deserving of concern and attention by policymakers, planners, and professionals.

THE CAREGIVER AS A FOCUS OF ATTENTION

For many years and in most programs, the focus of professional attention has been on the needs of the disabled elderly person. More recently, the caregivers have emerged from the background role of service-provider so that their own needs are being recognized and legitimated.

Professionals are confronted with the need to take a holistic approach to the family and to strike a delicate balance so that the needs of caregivers and care-recipients are met without disadvantaging one or the other. Most reports of respite programs, however, deal separately with effects of the service on

135

caregivers and care-recipients. A report from one project raised the issue of focus in terms of the allocation of scarce resources. Specifically, the question was the dilemma of the sponsoring agency in needing to choose between providing a bath for the patient and respite for the caregiver (Dixon-Bemis, 1986). In the same vein, as the first step in organizing a respite care program, it is important to consider whether the caregivers or the elderly are the target of services.

More subtle factors are also at work. It is not uncommon, for example, for caregivers to be reluctant to accept respite because the patient becomes (or might become) upset by a respite worker providing in-home care or by the environmental change involved in nursing home respite. The dilemma about who is the client is also expressed on the macro-level by such questions as how legislation is to be written or whose income (caregiver's or patient's) is to be considered in establishing eligibility criteria. Thus, the difficult task of effecting a true family approach is highlighted.

In targeting this controlled study of the effects of a respite care intervention to people with Alzheimer's disease, the focus was on those who care for an extremely disabled population. In comparison with national samples of disabled older people with all diagnoses (Kemper et al., 1986; Stone et al., 1987) the care-recipients in this program *needed* and *received* more help. Nevertheless, as in all studies of sources of assistance to the elderly, that help came preponderantly from the informal or family system, not from the formal system of government and agencies. The primary family caregivers had been providing care for an average of four years and were spending considerably more than the equivalent of a full-time job doing so—an average of almost 59 hours weekly. (Caregivers in the Channeling Demonstration were providing an average of about 42 hours weekly.) It is not surprising, therefore, that more than half of those over age 65 showed clinically significant depression, as did 42% of those under 65.

It is often overlooked that most caregivers for the disabled elderly receive some formal or informal respite that is not specifically labeled respite. This was, of course, the case with the caregivers in this study. Most of them had been receiving some such "unofficial" respite prior to the study either from family members or paid workers. The experimental intervention, then, represented additional respite for those who received it.

DEMAND FOR RESPITE CARE AND
LATENT DEMAND FOR OTHER SERVICES

Policymakers are often concerned lest the availability of subsidized formal services encourage family caregivers to reduce this help and unleash an unmanageable and costly demand. This was not the case in this study despite the fact that caregivers to Alzheimer's patients are a service-needy and high risk group. Although caregivers in the experimental group were offered, even encouraged, and in some instances urged to avail themselves of respite they obviously needed, only about half of them chose to use the service at all. Moreover, their requests were extremely modest and virtually all of them were willing to pay in accordance with their means.

The experimental group that was offered the respite intervention did increase its use of other community services slightly more than did the control group in the course of the treatment year. That outcome, after all, was one of the goals of the project. The central point is that (as in other studies) the added services did not substitute for family care. To emphasize: *The added respite and other services to which the experimental group of caregivers were referred did not encourage the caregivers to reduce or withdraw their own services.* In fact, caregivers in both the experimental and control groups *increased* the amount of help they provided during the year in which they were studied. That finding is not surprising in view of the inevitable downward trajectory in the functional capacities of Alzheimer's patients. The same pattern was evident with secondary family caregivers; even when additional help was forthcoming from the respite program, they too were steadfast in the amount of help they provided.

CONSUMER EVALUATION

Caregivers who received the experimental respite service gave that form of help a strong endorsement. Moreover, respite was named the most helpful and most wished for service by both the experimental and control groups. Multiple demonstrations of respite all over the country send the same message. Yet respite is often the least available service.

INSTITUTIONALIZATION, COMMUNITY-BASED CARE, AND COST OF RESPITE CARE

Although the caregivers were so overwhelmingly appreciative of respite and reported it to be so helpful, the service did not reduce rates of institutionalization greatly over the one year of the intervention, nor did it improve the caregivers' mental health. Explanations of these findings are straightforward.

It is not surprising that respite service prolonged community living of the patient only for a very modest period of time. No other respite program and no careful study of other attempts to reduce rates of nursing home admission via assessment, case management, or added services (e.g., Triage, Channeling) has accomplished that goal even with less impaired populations of older people. The precipitants of nursing home admissions are primarily the severe disabilities and heavy care requirements of the older people. These personal risk factors are in the main coupled with the lack of family caregivers or their exhaustion and inability to go on after long years of caregiving. Continued community care is often simply not possible unless services can actually substitute for the bulk of the sustained care needed on an ongoing daily and nightly basis. Such a plan requires virtually unlimited funds with which to employ three shifts of paid caregivers plus substitutes for staff vacation time, time off, and illness.

History shows that certain groups of older people are able to avoid institutional admissions. For example, intact and mildly impaired older people used to populate homes for the aged and county homes simply because they could not afford to live in the community, or because housing for the elderly (either with or without service supports built in) was nonexistent. Indeed, in the early part of this century, institutional care was seen as an alternative to what was called "outdoor relief"—that is, assistance in the community.

Apart from family care, the proven alternatives to institutional care for mildly impaired elderly are income maintenance and housing. One does well to remember that 50 years ago, half of all older people were totally dependent on their children economically and another 25% were receiving financial assistance from public or private agencies. With Social Security as a base, supplemented by pension plans and savings, only about 1.5% of older people now depend on their children for day-to-day financial support (Upp, 1982). Medicare has helped economically as well, preventing the aged from economic disaster as a result of acute illness. Housing for the elderly has come into being, some of which provides service supports. Despite their imperfections, together those programs have eliminated institutional admissions for the well and mildly disabled elderly so that now it is only the severely disabled who seek such care.

For the severely disabled such as Alzheimer's patients, it is inappropriate to advocate respite service and other community care services as a means of saving dollar costs and as "better" than institutional care. It has been shown definitively in all relevant studies that the dollar cost of community care for severely disabled old people is not less than nursing-home care. And for many old people and their families nursing-home care is the "better" plan. The cost issue really is a question of values. Is the dollar value the *only* value? Or, are the social costs—that is, the emotional and physical strains of caregivers—legitimate considerations? The literature is replete with documentation of such strains. In fact, for some caregivers the goal could well be to help them to do less rather than to continue at the same level of effort or to do more.

RESPITE CARE AND QUALITY OF CARE

On the set of outcome measures that evaluated caregiver well-being after the one year during which respite was offered to the experimental group, the control and experimental groups showed no significant differences. Yet, as in every other respite program (see Chapter 1 for review), the caregivers were overwhelmingly positive about the helpfulness of that form of service. It is not difficult to understand the failure of respite to improve "mental health." In this connection, the data bear repetition. Only 52% of those who were offered respite took advantage of the service. Of those, two-thirds chose in-home respite and received an average of 10.7 days of that service; 14% used institutional respite for periods of time ranging from 3 days to 3 weeks; and 4% used day care for an average of 17 days. Simple subtraction shows the number of days and nights during which they did *not* receive any service.

In addition, in this and all other studies of respite service, it was found that caregivers often view respite as an end-point service and fail to seek it until too late, when they are far along the path to severe stress and exhaustion. Some of the respite occurred a considerable time (up to 10 months) prior to the post-intervention evaluation at the end of the year. While a few hours or days of relief undoubtedly are helpful and provide a welcome rest, the caregivers then return to their arduous, stressful roles. And, because the inevitable trajectory is in the direction of more care and heavier care, those roles become ever more difficult. For respite to result in improvement in overall well-being and mental health of these caregivers, therefore, appears to be an unrealistic expectation.

Once again, then, values influence interpretation of the data. Is not respite service intrinsically "good" and needed if it provides caregivers with substitute care for the patient when the caregivers themselves are ill or hospitalized? If it allows them to go to family events? If it permits them to rest for a few hours or catch up on household and shopping chores? If it enables them to get out of the house for a short time? Or, must their overall mental health improve in order to justify the provision of service?

In short, the question is whether our values allow us to justify respite care simply because, as this study and all other studies have demonstrated, the caregivers needed it, wanted it, and reported that it had given them some welcome temporary relief.

RESPITE CARE AND SOCIAL POLICY

Social policy issues regarding the costs of respite services and how they are to be financed were not directly addressed by this research. Such issues regarding all types of long-term care services are being hotly debated by professionals, insurance companies and public policymakers, and a number of long-term care bills are currently before the U.S. Congress. A fundamental issue is whether such services (including respite) should be a universal entitlement of a social insurance program (as with Medicare), should be means tested (as with Medicaid), or should be purchased privately from insurance companies. It must be pointed out that the recent report by the Brookings Institution on methods for financing long-term care (Rivlin & Wiener, 1988) states that most people could not afford the private purchase of long-term care insurance. While social policy considerations regarding respite services do not differ appreciably from those governing all long-term care services, respite does present at least one dilemma if means testing is an option—whose income is to be tested, the elderly person's or the caregiver's?

THE VARIETIES OF RESPITE CARE

As there is more awareness of the need for respite service, other issues are arising such as the types of respite that should be available, the nature of the "model" (social or medical), and the kind of staffing (professional or volunteer). Experience with this project indicates clearly that there is no single answer to any of those questions. Disabled aged with Alzheimer's disease (virtually all of whom have other diagnoses as well) are extremely heterogeneous in the stage of the ailment and in their functioning levels and therefore in the kind of care they need. The kinds of respite services and the staffing patterns, therefore, must be keyed to those factors.

Allowing caregivers to choose the type of respite they wanted showed that the three forms of respite used in the project (in-home, day care, and institutional) did not substitute for each other nor were they in competition (see Chapter 5). Rather, they served different purposes for different people in different situations and who were at different points in their caregiving careers. Thus, all three types should be available to be used flexibly. Moreover, needs change over time and the choice of respite may change in response to the patient's and family's changing conditions and needs. Although caregivers chose in-home services much more often than day care or nursing home respite, that choice does not diminish the importance of the two latter services.

A footnote about the type of respite is the failure of the project to arrange care-sharing by unrelated caregivers. This is not surprising in view of the difficulties in caring for one, let alone two or more, such patients. In this connection, it is interesting to note that a major effort at effecting such care-sharing has been experiencing significant problems. Stone (1986) reports that the project—Elder Care Share in Michigan—had difficulty recruiting families to participate.

Overall, the project respite service was used for older patients and by those caregivers who were more burdened, who spent more time in caregiving, who were more depressed, and who at baseline expressed fewer positive emotions.

The characteristics of both caregivers and impaired elderly persons were associated with the forms of respite chosen and used. Day care often was not feasible for patients with disturbing behavioral symptoms and socially inappropriate behavior. Not only did such symptoms cause management problems at day care sites, but preparing and transporting them often posed seemingly insuperable barriers to the caregivers. Thus, these caregivers (who reported high subjective burdens) most often opted for in-home respite. Institutional respite was little used, but when it was, was chosen primarily for older patients by older caregivers who had been devoting the most time to caregiving at the outset of the study. Such families may be more vulnerable to emergencies that require total relief of the caregiver for a period of time.

STAFFING OF RESPITE PROGRAMS

Despite their helpfulness, all forms of respite can be improved. Attention is required to the quality of the various services involved. Staff training and behavior are major components of quality. There is consensus in the literature that programs should be under professional direction, with different types and levels of paid staff and volunteers being used in accordance with the characteristics of the population served. When attempted with extremely disabled patients, programs staffed solely by volunteers have failed.

As for the workers who perform the hands-on care, reports from the caregivers draw our attention to the home-health aides who provided much of the in-home respite care. The problems (high turnover, tardiness, unreliability, lack of skill, and inappropriate attitudes) described in this and in reports of other programs point to the need for training. Such workers, being dispersed in patients' homes, are more difficult to supervise than those who work in nursing homes and day care programs. Whether they are to be employed for in-home services or in nursing homes or day care centers, the recruitment, motivation, and training of a sufficient cadre of in-home workers is a major task for the decades ahead.

COMPONENTS OF A RESPITE PROGRAM

Although formal respite care is badly needed and in short supply, it is not a panacea needed or wanted by all caregivers. Nor is it a total solution to the problems inherent in family care, as experience and the case material presented in this book indicate. More often than not, the caregivers needed other services as well, both to enable them to use the respite as well as to complete the package of diverse services they required. For that reason, we reaffirm the conviction that any respite program must be accompanied by careful *assessment*; *caregiver education* about dementia and its management, and about the meaning and purpose of respite; *case management* to connect caregivers to other needed community services and to monitor the situations over time; and individual and family *counseling*. Equally important, if respite is not embedded in a total system of long-term care, at the least the program should have close linkages to other available services and be a component of a total system that provides continuity of care. The case management service is also needed to effect continuity of care—that is, to monitor changing needs so that service plans can be reformulated in response to changes in the patient or the family's situation.

Our experience shows that respite programs cannot be effective unless they are linked to or part of such a comprehensive system of long-term care services. First of all, families in need of respite are likely to have a constellation of other needs as well, and the use of respite more often than not requires the backup of other services. (Some such services are not officially called "respite," but often serve that purpose nonetheless—day care and in-home services from home-health aides or homemakers, for example.) Thus, a large number of referrals to other services were made by project staff. Second, to separate respite from the other components of a continuum of services would create additional fragmentation of an already fragmented system.

If a respite program is to link caregivers to other needed community services, those services must exist. A comprehensive system of long-term care does not exist at present. Services to maintain the disabled elderly and help their families to do so are in short supply, are uneven regionally, and their cost is often a barrier for families.

Even if public policy should permit the creation of all of the services needed, it would be an exercise in futility unless they were actually accessible to the families in need. Experience with the respite project once again illustrated the need for case management to deal with access problems. Some such problems are inherent in the organizational arrangements that families find confusing and defeating. The system is incoherent in that health services are multiple, parallel, overlapping and non-continuous; there are differing public streams of money, varied administrative arrangements, and a wide range of eligibility requirements (Brody & Woodfin, 1979).

EDUCATION ABOUT USING RESPITE CARE

The project also showed clearly that caregivers often do not know what respite service is. The nonuse and under-use of services by some of the neediest caregivers is a constant frustration to service workers. Reports about respite services, for example, including those for overburdened caregivers of Alzheimer's patients, consistently report that they are grossly underutilized despite concerted efforts at education and counseling. (Brody, Saperstein & Lawton, 1989; George 1988; Lawton, Brody et al., 1989; Lawton, Kleban et al., 1989; Montgomery, 1988; Saperstein & Brody, in press.)

Part of the problem is the lack of caregiver information and understanding about respite. That families are slow to use respite points to the crucial need to disseminate information about what respite is. This theme is reiterated in many descriptions of respite programs elsewhere (Montgomery, 1986, Packwood, 1980). Although the word "respite" is becoming familiar to professionals, it is not yet a concept familiar to the public as a treatment or a preventative measure. Caregivers are often reluctant to use respite services, and many view respite as an end-of-the-road service to be used when they are on the verge of breaking down. The demand for the service is almost invariably lower than anticipated (e.g., see Montgomery, 1986;

George & Gwyther, 1984). Caregivers in this project used the respite service judiciously and modestly, and were willing and eager to pay whatever they could. This experience calls into question the use of elaborate formulae and often humiliating procedures to determine expected payments. Without a subsidy, the threat of a long-term financial burden for respite care is a potent deterrent to use. Existing services and possible subsidies for them must be publicized and marketed if respite care is to reach the population to which it is targeted.

More subtle issues also impede service utilization and speak to the need for counseling or casework. As the case excerpts in this book illustrated, there are psychological barriers that inhibit some caregivers' use of needed services. (See, for example, Brody 1990.) In addition, the acceptability of services differs among older people with different socioeconomic and ethnic backgrounds and among individuals and families with diverse personalities and expectations. Therefore, whatever the label given to the process now most commonly referred to as "case management," it must include the enabling process called "counseling" or "casework."

There is a small but important proportion of caregivers for whom intensive counseling is essential to help them resolve psychological barriers that may prevent or inhibit use of the service. A noteworthy example is the subgroup of caregivers who require special help to extricate themselves from total, stressful caregiving situations that may be detrimental to their own health and well-being, to that of the patient, and sometimes to that of other family members. A different form of counseling—family group counseling—proved effective in selected situations, easing the burden of the primary caregiver and facilitating an orderly process of planning for the older person's care.

Because of the complex nature of the problems with which case managers deal, effective case management is a highly skilled knowledge- and value-based activity. It should not be seen solely as the mechanical manipulation or arrangement of service, but should include the offering of sensitive help with psychosocial issues. The blending of these activities cannot be carried out by untrained people, no matter how well-meaning they may be. Taken together, the complexity of the tasks involved and the high degree of skill required point clearly to the need for professional staff.

CONCLUSION

In conclusion, two matters bear repetition. First, respite is not, any more than any other single service, a panacea. Not all caregivers want or feel the need for that form of relief, and those who used the experimental respite program were the most vulnerable as indexed by burden, poor mental and physical health, and greater disability of the patient. We are left with the distressing finding that many are depressed and have other mental health symptoms. Certainly, respite service should be added to an inventory of readily available forms of help. Recognition that we can not do it all in alleviating the severe strains to which caregivers of Alzheimer's patients are subjected should not inhibit the search for additional ways to relieve that suffering.

Second, the focus of this book on caregivers was not meant to obscure the needs of the patients themselves for care and treatment. Attention must be paid to the needs of the uniquely disadvantaged people who are afflicted with Alzheimer's disease, especially those who have no family to provide the devoted, arduous care so amply demonstrated by the caregivers we studied and their peers everywhere.

References

Adult Services, Social Services Division. (1984). *Respite care services.* Report to the Department of Human Services, State of Minnesota, August.

Archbold, P. (1978). Impact of caring for an ill elderly parent of the middle-aged or elderly offspring caregiver. Paper presented at the 31st Annual Meeting of the Gerontological Society, Dallas, TX.

Baltimore/Central Maryland Alzheimer's Association. (1989). Caregivers Assistance Respite Program Pamphlet. Baltimore: Author.

Bradburn, N.M. (1969). *The structure of psychological well being.* Chicago, IL: Aldine Publihing Co.

Brody, E.M. (1981). Women in the middle and family help to older people. *The Gerontologist, 21,* 471–480.

Brody, E.M. (1985). The role of the family in nursing homes: Implications for research and public policy. In M.S. Harper & B. Lebowitz, (Eds.), *Mental illness in nursing homes: Agenda for research.* (pp. 234–264) National Institute of Mental Health. Washington, DC: U.S. Government Printing Office, 234–264.

Brody, E.M. (1987). The family at risk. In E. Light & B. Lebowitz, (Eds.), *Alzheimer's disease treatment and family stress: Direc-*

149

tions for research. National Institute of Mental Health, Washington, DC.

Brody, E.M. (1990). *Women in the middle: Their parent care years,* New York: Springer Publishing Co.

Brody, E.M., Dempsey, N.P., & Pruchno, R.A. (1990). Mental health of sons and daughters of the institutionalized aged: Mental Health Effects. *The Gerontologist, 30,* 212–219.

Brody, E.M., Johnsen, P.T., & Fulcomer, M.C. (1982). Women in the middle and care of the dependent elderly—Final Report on AoA Grant #90-AR-2174.

Brody, E.M., Kleban, M.H., Johnsen, P.T., Hoffman, C., & Schoonover, C.B. (1987). Work status and parent care: A comparison of four groups of women. *The Gerontologist, 27,* 201–208.

Brody, E.M., Kleban, M.H., Lawton, M.P., & Silverman, H. (1971). Excess disabilities of mentally impaired aged: Impact of individualized treatment. *The Gerontologist, 11,* 124–133.

Brody, E.M., Lawton, M.P., & Liebowitz, B. (1984). Senile dementia: Public policy and adequate institutional care. *American Journal of Public Health, 74,* 1381–1383.

Brody, S.J., Poulshock, S.W., & Masciocchi, C.T. (1978). The family caring unit: A major consideration in the long-term support system. *Gerontologist, 18,* 556–561.

Brody, E.M., Saperstein, A.R., & Lawton, M.P. (1989). A multi-service respite program for caregivers of Alzheimer's patients. *Journal of Gerontological Social Work, 14* (1/2), 41–74.

Brody, S.J. & Woodfin, A.B. (1979). *Long-term support systems: An analysis of health systems agency plans.* Philadelphia, PA, National Health Care Management Center, University of Pennsylvania.

California Department of Mental Health. (1987). Family survival project for brain damaged adults. Final Report of Second-Year Progress of a State Pilot Project, San Francisco, CA.

Cantor, M.H. (1980). Caring for the frail elderly: Impact on family, friends and neighbors. Paper presented at the 33rd Annual Meeting of the Gerontological Society of America, San Diego, CA.

Capitman, J. (1989). Policy and program options in community oriented long-term care. In M.P. Lawton (Ed.) *Annual review of gerontology and geriatrics,* Vol. 9. New York: Springer Publishing Co.

Cohen, D., & Eisdorfer, C. (1986). *The loss of self: A family resource for the care of Alzheimer's disease and related disorders*. New York: W.W. Norton.

Comptroller General of the United States. (1977a). Home health—the need for a national policy to better provide for the elderly. Report to the Congress. U.S. General Accounting Office, Washington, DC.

Comptroller General of the United States. (1977b). *The well-being of older people in Cleveland, Ohio*. U.S. General Accounting Office, #RD-77-70, Washington, DC, April 19.

Connecticut Department of Health Services. (1983). Respite Care Demonstration Program. Community Nursing and Home Health Division, Office of Public Health, Hartford, CT.

Cornoni-Huntley, J.C., Foley, D.J., White, L.R., Suzman, R., Berkman, L.F., Evans, D.A., & Wallace, R.B. (1985). Epidemiology of disability in the oldest old: Methodologic issues and preliminary findings. *Milbank Memorial Fund Quarterly, 63*, 350–376.

Crossman, L., London, C., & Barry, C. (1981). Older women caring for disabled spouses: A model for supportive services. *The Gerontologist, 21*, 464–470.

Crozier, M.C. (1982, September/October). Respite care keeps elders at home longer. *Perspective on Aging*, 11–22.

Danis, B.G. (1978). Stress in individuals caring for ill elderly relatives. Paper presented at the 31st Annual Meeting of the Gerontological Society, Dallas, TX.

Deimling, G.T., & Bass, D.M. (1986). Symptoms of mental impairment among elderly adults and their effects on family caregivers. *Journal of Gerontology, 41*, 778–784.

Dixon-Bemis, J. (1986). Respite as a continuum of services: The Arizona approach. In R. Montgomery & J. Prothero (Eds.), *Developing respite services for the elderly*, (pp. 50–60). Seattle: University of Washington Press.

Doty, P., Liu, K., & Wiener, J. (1985) An overview of long-term care. *Health Care Financing Review, 6*, 69–78.

Dunn, L. (1986). Senior Respite Care Program. *Pride Institute Journal of Long Term Care*, Summer, 5, 7–12.

Dunn, R.B., MacBeath, L., & Robertson, D. (1983). Respite admissions and the disabled elderly. *Journal of the American Geriatrics Society, 31*, 613–616.

Ellis, V. (1986). Respite in an institution. In R. Montgomery &

J. Prothero (Eds.), *Developing respite services for the elderly* (pp. 61–68). Seattle: University of Washington Press.

Ellis, V., & Wilson, D. (1983). Respite Care in the nursing home unit of a veterans hospital. *American Journal of Nursing,* October, 1433–1434.

Evans, E.M. (1985). Multilingual Volunteers Help Respite Program. *The Kansas Capital Areas Chapter, American Red Cross, 1,* (3).

Fengler, A.P., & Goodrich, N. (1979) Wives of elderly disabled men: The hidden patients. *The Gerontologist, 19,* 175–183.

Fox, P.D., & Clauser, S.B. (1980). Trends in nursing home expenditures: Implications for aging policy. *Health Care Financing,* Review/Fall, 65–70.

Fulton, J.P., & Katz, S. (1986). Characteristics of the disabled elderly and implications for rehabilitation. In S.J. Brody, & G.E. Ruff (Eds.), *Aging & rehabilitation-Advances in the state of the art,* (pp. 36–46). New York: Springer Publishing Co.

George, L.K. (1984). The burden of caregiving: How much? What kinds? For whom? *Advances in Research,* Duke University, Center for the Study of Aging and Human Development, Vol. 8, No. 2.

George, L.K. (1984) The Dynamics of Caregiver Burden, Final Report submitted to the AARP Andrus Foundation, December.

George, L.K. (1986). Respite care: Evaluating a strategy for easing caregiver burden. *Center Reports on Advances in Research, 10,* No. 2, pp. 1–7. Duke University Center, for the Study of Aging and Human Development.

George, L.K. (1988). Why won't caregivers use community services? Paper presented at the Annual Meeting of the Gerontological Society of America, Washington, DC.

George, L.K., & Gwyther, L.P. (1984). Respite care: A strategy for easing caregiver burden, Abstract. Duke University, Center for Aging and Human Development by the AARP/Andrus Foundation.

Gibson, M.J. (1982). An international update on family care of the ill elderly. *Ageing International, 9,* 11–14.

Gold, M. (1986). Parents of the older developmentally disabled look at the future. *Brookdale Center on Aging Newsletter,* Hunter College/CUNY, 8(5).

Grad, J., & Sainsbury, P. (undated). An Evaluation of the Effects of Caring for the Aged at Home. Mimeo.

Grad, J., & Sainsbury, P. (1966). Problems of caring for the mentally ill at home. *Proceedings of the Royal Society of Medicine*, Section of Psychiatry, *59*, 20–23.

Grana, J.M. (1983). Disability allowances for long-term care in Western Europe and the United States. *International Social Security Review*, February, 207–221.

Gurland, B.J., & Cross, P.S. (1986). Public health perspectives or clinical memory testing of Alzheimer's disease and related disorders. In L.W. Poon (Eds.), *Clinical memory asessment of older adults* (pp. 11–20). Washington, DC: American Psychological Association.

Gurland, B., Dean, L., Gurland, R., & Cook, D. (1978). Personal time dependency in the elderly of New York City: Findings from the U.S.-U.K. cross-national geriatric community study. In *Dependency in the Elderly of New York City* (pp. 9–45). Community Council of Greater New York.

Gwyther, L., & Ballard, E. (1988). In-home respite care: Guidelines for training respite workers serving memory impaired adults. Durham, NC: Duke University Center on Aging.

Gwyther, L., & Ballard, E. (1988). In-home respite care: Guidelines for programs serving family caregivers for memory impaired adults. Durham, NC: Duke University Center for Aging.

Hevern, W. (1985). Personal communications re: Care Tenders Home Health Agency, Louisville, KY.

Hildebrandt, E.D. (1983). Respite care in the home. *American Journal of Nursing*, October, 1428–1430.

Hornbaker, A. (1983). Respite care program will give families of elderly needed break. *The Cincinnati Enquirer*, September 11, E-10 Tempo.

Horowitz, A. (1985). Family caregiving to the frail elderly. In C. Eisdorfer, M.P. Lawton, & G.L. Maddox, (Eds.), *Annual review of gerontology and geriatrics*, Vol. 5 (pp. 194–246). New York: Springer Publishing Co.

Horowitz, A., & Dobrof, R. (1982). The Role of Families in Providing Long-Term Care to the Frail and Chronically Ill Elderly Living in the Community. Final Report submitted to the Health Care Financing Administration, Department of Health and Human Services.

Katzman, R., & Karasu, T.B. (1975). Differential diagnosis of dementia. In W.S. Fields (Eds.), *Neurological and sensory disorders in the elderly* (pp. 103–134). New York: Stratton International Medical Book Corp.

Kemper, P., Applebaum, R., & Harrigan, M. (1987). Community care demonstrations: What have we learned? *Health Care Financing Review, 8,* 87–100.

Kemper, P., Brown, R.S., Carcagno, G.J., et al. (1986). The evaluation of the National Long Term Care Demonstration: Final Report. Contact No. HHS-100-80-0157. Prepared for Department of Health & Human Services. Princeton, NJ: Mathematica Policy Research.

Kiecolt-Glaser, J.K., Glasser, R., Shuttleworth, E.C., Dyer, C.S., Ozroclsi, P., & Speicher, C.E. (1987). Chronic stress and immunity in family caregivers of Alzheimer's disease victims, *Psychosomatic Medicine, 49,* 523–535.

Kleban, M.H., Brody, E.M., & Lawton, M.P. (1971). Personality traits in the mentally-impaired aged and their relationship to improvements in current functioning. *The Gerontologist, 11,* 134–140.

Lang, A., & Brody, E.M. (1983). Characteristics of middle-aged daughters and help to their elderly mothers. *Journal of Marriage and the Family, 45,* 193–202.

Lawton, M.P. (1983). The dimensions of wellbeing. *Experimental Aging Research, 9,* 65–72.

Lawton, M.P., Brody, E.M., & Saperstein, A.R. (1989). A controlled study of respite service for caregivers of Alzheimer's patients. *The Gerontologist, 29,* 8–16.

Lawton, M.P., Brody, E.M., Saperstein, A., & Grimes, M. (1989). Respite services for caregivers: Research findings for service planning. *Home Health Care Services Quarterly, 10,* 5–32.

Lawton, M.P., Kleban, M.H., Moss, M., Rovine, M., & Glicksman, A. (1989). Meauring caregiving appraisal. *Journal of Gerontology: Psychological Sciences, 3,* 61–71.

Lawton, M.P. & Lawton, F.G. (Eds.) (1965). *Mental impairment in the aged.* Philadelphia: Philadelphia Geriatric Center.

Lazarus, R.S., & Folkman, S. (1984). *Stress appraisal and coping.* New York: Springer Publishing Co.

Litman, T.J. (1971). Health care and the family: A three-generational analysis. *Medical Care, 9,* 67–81.

Mace, N., & Rabins, P. (1981). *The 36-Hour Day: A family guide to caring for persons with Alzheimer's disease, related dementing illness and memory loss in late life.* Baltimore, MD: Johns Hopkins University Press.

McGuane, P. (1989). Cooperative approaches to respite care: Three community models. Paper presented at the Exemplary Respite Care for Alzheimer's Patients and Families, Cambridge, MA.

Meltzer, J.W. (1982, June). Respite care: An emerging family support service. The Center for the Study of Social Policy. Washington, DC.

Miller, D.B., Gulle, N., & McCue, F. (1986). The realities of respite for families, clients, and sponsors. *The Gerontologist, 26,* 467–470.

Montgomery, R.J. (1986). Researching respite: Beliefs, facts, & questions. In R. Montgomery & J. Prothero (Eds.), *Developing respite services for the elderly* (pp. 18–32). Seattle: University of Washington Press.

Montgomery, R.J. (1988). Respite care: Lessons from a controlled design study. *Health Care Financing Review, 9* (suppl.), 133–138.

Montgomery, R.J., & Borgatta, E.F. (1985) Family support project—Final report on AOA Grant #90AM0046.

Montgomery, R.J., & Prothero, J. (Eds.) (1986). *Developing respite services for the elderly.* Seattle & London: University of Washington Press.

Mosely, E. (1983). Personal communications re: Respite care program. Division of Aging. Kansas, MO.

Moss, M., & Kurland, P. (1979). Family visiting with institutionalized mentally impaired aged. *Journal of Gerontological Social Work, 1,* 271–278.

Munson, J. (1983). Personal communication re: Adult respite care project. Delaware County Office for the Aging, Media.

National Center for Health Statistics. (May 14, 1987). E. Hing: Use of nursing homes by the elderly, Preliminary data from the 1985 National Nursing Home Survey. *Advance Data From Vital and Health Statistics.* No. 135, DHHS Pub. No. (PHS)87–1250. Public Health Service, Hyattsville, MD.

National Council of Catholic Women (NCCW). (1983). Respite: A way to ease the burden. Perspective on Aging, July/Aug, 9.

Newman, S.J. (1976) Housing adjustments of older people: A report from second phase. Ann Arbor, MI: University of Michigan, Institute for Social Research.

Noelker, L.S. & Poulshock, S.W. (1982) The effects on families of caring for impaired elderly in residence. Final Report, AoA Grant #90-AR-2112, Benjamin Rose Institute, Cleveland, OH, October.

Packwood, T. (1980) Supporting the family: A study of the organization and implications of hospital provision of holiday relief for families caring for dependents at home. *Social Science and Medicine, 14A,* 613–620.

Palmer, H.C. (1983). The alternatives question. In R.J. Vogel, & H.C. Palmer, (Eds.), *Long-term care, perspectives from research and demonstrations* (pp. 255–305). Health Care Financing Administration, U.S. DHHS.

Palmer, B. (1981). Community care for the elderly. Instructional material for determining ability to pay and assessment fees. Department of Health and Rehabilitative Services, Tallahassee, FL.

Pfeffer, R.I., Afifi, A.A., & Chance, J.M. (1987). Prevalence of Alzheimer's disease in a retirement community. *American Journal of Epidemiology, 125,* 420–436.

Quinn, T., & Crabtree, J. (1987) *How to start a respite service for people with Alzheimer's and their families.* New York: Brookdale Foundation.

Rabbit, W. (1986). The New York respite demonstration project. In R. Montgomery & J. Prothero (Eds.), *Developing respite services for the elderly* (pp. 33–49). Seattle: University of Washington Press.

Radloff, L.S. (1977). The CES-D Scale: A self-report depression scale for research in the general population. *Applied Psychological Measurement, 1,* 385–401.

Report on the Advisory Panel on Alzheimer's Disease. (1989). Submitted to the Congress of the United States, to the Secretary, U.S. Department of Health and Human Services, and to the Council on Alzheimer's Disease, U.S. Department of Health and Human Services.

Respite Care Demonstration Projects. (1986). A Report to the 1986 Legislature. Bureau of Aging and Adult Services, Community Services Division, Olympia, WA, January.

Rivlin, A.M., & Wiener, J.M. (1988) *Caring for the disabled elderly: Who will pay?* Washington, DC: The Brookings Institute.

Robertson, D., Griffiths, R.A., & Cosin, L.Z. (1977). A community-based continuing care program for the elderly disabled. *Journal of Gerontology, 32,* 334–339.

Rowland, R.H. (1985). Respite Care. Commonwealth of Massachusetts, Executive Office of Elder Affairs, Boston, MA, March 22.

Russell, S.L. (1983). Respite Care Homes Program begins in Baltimore

County. Baltimore County Department of Social Services, Towson, MD.

Safford, F. (1986). *Caring for the mentally impaired elderly: A family guide.* New York: Henry Holb and Co.

Sands, D., & Suziki, T. (1983). Adult day care for Alzheimer's patients and their families. *The Gerontologist, 23,* 21–23.

Saperstein, A.R., & Brody, E.M. (in press). What types of respite services do family caregivers of Alzheimer's patients want? *Aging Magazine.*

Scharlach, A., & Frenzel, C. (1986). An evaluation of institution-based respite care. *The Gerontologist, 26,* 77–82.

Seltzer, B., Fabiszewaski, K., Brown, J., & Lyon, P. (1985). A multidisciplinary team approach to the outpatient with Alzheimer's disease. Paper presented at Annual Meeting of the Gerontological Society of America, New Orleans, LA.

Seltzer, B., Rheaume, Y., Volicer, L., Fabiszewski, K., Lyon, P., Brown, J., & Volicer, B. (1988). The short-term effects of in-hospital respite on the patient with Alzheimer's Disease. *The Gerontologist, 28,* 121–124.

Shanas, E. (1961). *Family relationships of older people.* Health Information Foundation, Research Series 20. University of Chicago, Chicago, IL.

Spence, D.L., & Miller, D.B. (1985/1986). Family respite for the elderly Alzheimer's patient. *Journal of Gerontological Social Work, 9,* 101–112.

Stehouwer, J. (1968). The household and family relations of old people. In E. Shanas, P. Townsend, D. Wedderburn, H. Friis, P. Milhoj, & J. Stehouwer, (Eds.), *Old people in three industrial societies* (pp. 177–226). New York: Atherton Press.

Stone, R. (1986). Aging in the Eighties—Use of community services, preliminary data from the Supplement on Aging to the National Health Interview Survey: United States, Jan.–June 1984, *National Center for Health Statistic Advanced Data From Vital and Health Statistics,* No. 124 (DHHS Pub. No. (PHS) 86-1250), Public Health Service.

Stone, R., Cafferata, G.L., & J. Sangl. (1987). Caregivers of the frail elderly: A national profile. *The Gerontologist, 27,* 616–626.

Sussman, M.B. (1976). The family life of old people. In R.H. Binstock, & E. Shanas (Eds.), *Handbook of aging and the social sciences.* New York: Van Nostrand Reinhold.

Texas Department of Human Resources. (1982). Community Care Demonstration Projects, Evaluation Report. Office of Research Demonstration and Evaluation, Austin, TX, March.

U.S. Congress, Office of Technology Assessment. (1987). *Losing a million minds: Confronting the tragedy of Alzheimer's disease and other dementias*, OTA-BA-323. Washington, DC: U.S. Government Printing Office.

U.S. Department of Health and Human Services, National Center for Health Statistics. (1981). Characteristics of Nursing Home Residents, Health Status, and Care Received: National Nursing Home Survey, United States, May-December 1977. *Vital Health Statistics*, Series 13, No. 51, DHHS Pub. No. (PHS)81-1712.

U.S. Public Health Service. (1972). *Home Care for Persons Aged 55 and Over in the U.S.*, July 1966–June 1968, *Vital and Health Statistics*, Series 10, No. 73, DHEW, July.

Upp, M. (1982). A look at the economic status of the aged then and now. *Social Security Bulletin, 45,* 16–22.

Vintage, Inc. (1985). *Family Handbook of Family to Family. A Respite Co-op.* Pittsburgh, PA: Vintage.

Weissert, W.G. (1985). Seven reasons why it is so difficult to make community based long-term care cost effective. *HSR: Health Services Research, 20,* No. 4, 423–431.

White, J., & Ehrlich, P. (1988). Time Off Promotes Strength (TOPS): A model integrating practice and research in respite service. Paper presented at the 41st Annual Meeting of the Gerontological Society of America, San Francisco, CA.

Whitfield, S. (1981). Report to the General Assembly on the Family Demonstration Program. State of Maryland, Office on Aging, August.

Wisconsin Department of Health and Social Services. (1983). Respite Care Projects, Final Report. Division of Community Services, Office on Aging, Madison, WI.

Yocom, B. (1982). Respite care options for families caring for the frail elderly. Pacific Northwest Long-Term Care Center, University of Washington, Seattle, WA.

Zarit, S.H., Reever, K.E., & Bach-Peterson, J. (1980). Relatives of the impaired elderly: Correlation of feelings of burden. *The Gerontologist, 20,* 649–655.

Zawadski, R.T. (Guest Ed.) (1983). Community-based systems of long term care. *Home Health Care Services Quarterly,* (3/4).

Zimmer, A.H., & Mellor, M.J. (1981). Caregivers make the difference

(The Natural Supports Program). Community Service Society, New York, September.

Zimmer, A.H., & Sainer, J.S. (1978). Strengthening the family as an information support for their aged: Implications for social policy and planning. Paper presented at the 31st Annual Meeting of the Gerontological Society, Dallas, TX.

Index

161

RC523 .L38 1991   c.1
Lawton, M. Powell (M   100107 000
Respite for caregivers of Alzh

3 9310 00088837 8
GOSHEN COLLEGE-GOOD LIBRARY